Cafeteria Management for Hospitals

Faisal A. Kaud
R. Paul Miller
Robert F. Underwood

Y 10 2

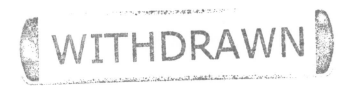

American Hospital Association
840 North Lake Shore Drive
Chicago, Illinois 60611

Library of Congress Cataloging in Publication Data

Kaud, Faisal A.
   Cafeteria management for hospitals.

   Bibliography: p.
   1. Hospitals—Food service—Management. I. Miller,
R. Paul. II. Underwood, Robert F. III. Title.
RA975.5.D5K38 1982   647'.95   82-11397
ISBN 0-87258-379-1

AHA Catalog No. 046200

©1982 by the
American Hospital Association
840 North Lake Shore Drive
Chicago, Illinois 60611

CONTENTS

LIST OF FIGURES

PREFACE

Cafeteria Management for Hospitals has been prepared primarily for food service administrators who are responsible for the management of public feeding in a health care institution. Hospital food service administrators are constantly challenged by the rapidly changing health care financial environment and by the rising costs of food, labor, and material in a volatile marketplace. These conditions make a significant impact on the health care provider and, as a result, the management and control of costs have become increasingly important in hospital food service management.

This book deals exclusively with hospital food service to nonpatients and is intended to give food service administrators the information needed to manage the nonpatient food service area in the most professional manner possible. It outlines the necessary tools for operating the hospital cafeteria in a predetermined manner and for providing customer satisfaction, employee productivity, and the achievement of the institution's financial objectives.

It is hoped that food service administrators and students in the field of institutional food management will find *Cafeteria Management for Hospitals* a helpful resource for the successful management of a hospital food service cafeteria in particular and public food service in general.

The authors gratefully acknowledge the support of the American Society for Hospital Food Service Administrators of the American Hospital Association in developing and preparing this publication. They also express their thanks for the assistance provided by Bonnie B. Miller, former senior staff specialist, and Mary R. DeMarco, senior staff specialist, Office of Human Resources—Personal Membership Services, American Hospital Association. Editorial services were provided by Beryl Dwight, staff editor, Book Department, under the direction of Dorothy Saxner, director, Division of Books and Newsletters, American Hospital Association.

Faisal A. Kaud is administrator, food service, environmental service, and materials management, University of Wisconsin Hospital and Clinics, Madison; R. Paul Miller is director of food service, Greenwich Hospital Association, Greenwich, Connecticut; and Robert F. Underwood is director, food and nutrition services, Maine Medical Center, Portland.

Part A. Management Functions

CHAPTER 1
INTRODUCTION TO PART A

Food service administrators, dietitians, and the majority of employees in a hospital food service department are employed for one primary reason—the proper nutritional care of patients. In addition, however, food service personnel have responsibilities to provide food to such nonpatient areas and functions as meetings, parties, a coffee shop, vending machines, meals on wheels, and a cafeteria. The cafeteria may account for a very small percentage of the total services rendered by the food service department, or it may serve more people and handle a greater volume of food than the patient area of the department does. Whatever the size of the cafeteria, the operation of an efficient, productive, and enjoyable cafeteria will be helped by the guidelines presented here.

The cafeteria may be easier to visualize as a business operation than the patient service area, because cash is actually exchanged and management is able to greet customers at their tables just as in a commercial restaurant. In addition, because the food service department is directly exchanging food and service for money and because many customers are a semicaptive audience for the duration of their careers at the hospital, the cafeteria must be managed in an efficient and effective manner.

In part A, 12 major concerns that must be recognized and dealt with in any well managed hospital cafeteria are discussed. These concerns are general in nature and apply to every hospital cafeteria, although the exact method of implementation will vary from institution to institution. Where possible, more than one method of approaching a subject has been given so that the food service administrator can choose the most appropriate one. The information is, by design, easily adaptable to almost any operation and is supplemented by references that will provide more choices for readers to apply to a specific operation. For example, although the meat specifications used as an illustration in the text may be applicable to many hospital cafeterias, reference is also made to the National Association of Meat Purveyors' *Meat Buyers' Guide* and the U.S. Department of Agriculture's *Institutional Meat Purchase Specifications* (see Bibliography), publications that will give enough additional information to develop suitable meat specifications for any hospital cafeteria.

CHAPTER 2
MENU PLANNING AND DEVELOPMENT

A customer-oriented menu is the first step toward successful management of the hospital cafeteria. A customer-oriented menu represents three points of view: that of the customer, who enjoys good dining; that of the employee, who prepares the food and serves it attractively; and that of the manager, who accounts for operating the cafeteria in an efficient and cost-effective manner.

The food service administrator recognizes the importance of certain operational elements and must have the necessary knowledge to (1) plan a profitable menu; (2) purchase high-quality food at economical prices; (3) receive and store food supplies properly; (4) control the issuing of food, (5) prepare and process foods according to standard recipes, standard cooking and processing procedures, and standard quality; (6) serve foods attractively and in standard portion sizes; and (7) account for sales of food. The food service administrator knows that the menu determines the foods to be purchased, the equipment and personnel needed, the work schedules, the level of supervision, and the cost of operation.

PREPLANNING CONSIDERATIONS

Before actually writing menus, the menu planner takes into consideration certain factors that are essential to a successful meal plan. One factor is a knowledge of the customers to be served—their food habits as evidenced by their racial, regional, and religious background; their nutritional needs based on age, sex, and occupation; and the size of the group. Another factor is awareness of the resources required to provide an attractive and nutritious meal. These resources include the number of food service employees and their skills and capabilities; the physical facility of the cafeteria, including the type and layout of equipment; and the funds allocated for food and personnel costs. In addition, an understanding is needed of such external influences on meal planning as the season, the climate, the availability of foods, and prevailing food fads.

KNOWLEDGE OF THE CUSTOMERS

- *Food habits.* Customer habits play an important role in determining the menu to be offered, the type of food required, and the personnel and equipment needed to prepare the desired menu. The racial, regional, and religious preferences of customers to be served are significant factors to

consider in planning a menu. For example, regional food habits within the United States are distinctive, and each set of habits is extremely popular in its own region. Hominy grits, black-eyed peas, mustard and
- successful menu in a southern hospital cafeteria and might fail absolutely to please the customer of a New England hospital cafeteria. Thus, the menu planner should recognize regional preferences and habits and prepare a menu to incorporate the specific wishes and needs of the customer.
- *Nutritional needs.* The nutritional requirements of the hospital cafeteria customers are an important consideration in meal planning. One of the objectives of a health care institution is to enhance the learning opportunity of its employees and visitors through active participation in personal nutritional awareness. This objective is accomplished by offering classes and reading material to help customers make food purchases from the cafeteria based on informed decisions. The menu planner should recognize the importance of this need and provide adequate food variety to enable customers to make the appropriate decision.

NECESSARY RESOURCES

- *Personnel.* The menu planner is fully aware of the significant impact of the menu on food production and service personnel. The menu dictates the number of employees needed, the level of skill required, and the hours of preparation necessary to produce and serve the menu.
- *Equipment.* The menu requirements should be supported by the appropriate and necessary equipment in order to produce the menu in an attractive fashion. In addition, it is essential that the menu be designed to equalize equipment use and employee work loads.
- *Availability of budgetary funds.* A full understanding of the total costs associated with the production and service of a particular menu is essential. It is equally important that the total menu costs be within the health care institution's budget. The food service administrator has the responsibility to account for hospital cafeteria costs and to monitor them closely.

All menu planning should proceed from the premise that the primary purpose of any hospital cafeteria is to plan, prepare, and serve attractive, flavorful, and nourishing meals at a cost consistent with the policy of the health care institution. To prepare for the details of menu planning, preliminary considerations of menu mechanics, menu analysis, and menu balancing should be addressed.

MENU MECHANICS

Menu mechanics refers to a number of procedures that require certain decisions to be made in advance to ensure that planning proceeds in an orderly fashion. Decisions need to be made on the number of days to be planned at one time, whether or not to use cycle menus, the number of choices to be offered, and the form for writing the menus. The procedures based on these decisions are as follows:

1. *Planning cycle.* The planning cycle is the number of days for which

menus are planned at one time. Many menu planners prefer to use an 8-day, 10-day, or 12-day period because it helps to eliminate the possibility of serving the same food item on the same day each week.

✛ 2. *Cycle menu.* A cycle menu consists of sets of menus that are rotated at definite intervals. Hospital cafeteria menus are planned for two or three weeks or more, at the end of which time the same menus are repeated. In many cases, the hospital cafeteria cycle menu is planned in conjunction with the patient menu to facilitate production work load and to maximize the efficient use of personnel and equipment.

3. *Menu pattern.* The menu pattern is an outline of the types of food items to be included in each meal, indicating the extent to which these items are decided on before menus are planned. For example, the menu pattern for a hospital cafeteria for a lunch meal may consist of one soup, one chili, six entrees, one hot sandwich, two potatoes, two vegetables, five salads, six desserts, and six cold sandwiches.

4. *Menu form.* A menu form is designed to capture basic menu pattern information in order to facilitate the planning of the menu in an organized manner. One simple form lists the types of menu items that must be planned in the left-hand column and provides space for the menu items to be written in as they are chosen (see figure 2A). Such a form provides an easily followed reference as the cycle grows to full length.

MENU ANALYSIS

A careful study of sales information is important to determine the precise preferences of the customer. This study may be accomplished by gathering sales information each time a particular menu is sold. This information can be manually maintained or obtained from electronic cash registers or other data-gathering equipment. The analysis of sales will show what the customers want and the prices they are willing to pay. Once the most popular items have been determined, a method of rotating the menu will have to be decided on in order to provide the customer with variety and to even the production work load on personnel and equipment.

MENU BALANCING

The menu planner requires a thorough knowledge of nutrition, food production, accounting, and management in order to balance the menu in an attractive manner. To excel in balancing the menu, the menu planner must be able to:

1. Select the entrees so as to achieve a variety of meat, fowl, and seafood.
2. Feature popular food items on "Today's Special."
3. Select the juices, soups, vegetables, salads, and desserts to complement the entree. Offer a variety of color in the juices, a heavy and a light soup, a variety of texture and colors in the vegetables, a variety of salads with a choice of four or more dressings (including a low-calorie dressing), and a variety of desserts.
4. Provide an appropriate approach to pricing the menu. Offer a balanced price between the high and low cost for items to ensure the attainment of a high average check.
5. Consider the following food characteristics when placing a food item on

the menu: color, texture, consistency, arrangement, shape or form, size portion, and the overall look of the food combination.

6. Consider the season and the climate, which have a direct effect on the type of menu items that would be popular with customers. Provide appropriate food when in season.

7. Identify and describe menu items accurately. Misleading information or misrepresentation of facts should not appear on the menu. Restaurant associations have conducted voluntary programs for their members advising them to watch out for these possibly misleading words: *natural* food, *fresh* shrimp cocktails, *maple* syrup, *choice* steaks, and *homemade* cheesecake. Some states have legislation pending and others have ordinances or guidelines, but all food service administrators have the same eleventh commandment governing their lives: Thou shalt not misrepresent thy offering to thy customer, be it in product identification (Is your chicken salad actually turkey, your 16-oz steak actually 12 oz?), point of origin (Are your Idaho potatoes from Washington?), method of preparation (Are your fried-in-butter scallops actually deep-fried in oil?), or pictorial description (Is your strawberry shortcake made with sliced strawberries when the menu photo depicts whole ones?). Merchandising expressions such as "roast beef piled high on rye," "our own special blend of coffee," "milk-fed veal," and "a generous portion of prime rib" are all examples that must be checked for accuracy. There are other avenues to tread, however; a state restaurant association advises, for instance, the substitution of the word *chilled* for *fresh* if frozen shrimp are served; the same may be said for describing canned fruit or fruit juices.

8. Study the competition in these areas: type of consumer, menu variety, prices, type of service, hours of operation, and decor. The answer to the following questions may assist the food service administrator in formulating a competitive strategy to improve the hospital cafeteria revenues:

   a. What kind of customers is your competitor attracting? What time? What day of the week?

   b. Is there much competition? Is there very little competition?

   c. Are you competing with fast food restaurants or restaurant-bars?

   d. How much of the local population do you think you attract or should attract with your menu?

   e. Are you really catering to the needs of your customers at the right times in the right way and at the right prices?

   f. Where are you lacking?

   g. What kind of business are you missing out on? Can you correct the deficiency?

   h. Are you staying open too long, or are you closing too early and missing out on late business?

This chapter has emphasized the approaches and strategies to be taken in developing an effective customer-oriented menu. They will provide a solid foundation on which the food service administrator can establish standards and procedures to manage the hospital cafeteria in the most efficient manner.

Figure 2A.
Cycle Menu Planner

Item		Day	Day	Day	Day
Lunch					
Soup					
Hot-plate special					
Special sandwich					
Vegetable					
Vegetable					
Vegetable					
Salad					
Dessert					
Dinner					
Chef's special					
Dietitian's special					
Vegetable					
Vegetable					
Vegetable					
Salad					
Dessert					

CHAPTER 3
ESTABLISHING STANDARDS

Each time a customer orders an item, it should meet established expectations of taste, quality, size, and appearance consistent with every previous offering of that item to the customer. To provide that consistency, standards for purchasing, recipes, portions, and service must be established.

When the menu is originally planned, the food service administrator, dietitian, or menu planner envisions each product as he or she expects it to be served and as it relates to the other products being served at the same time. The hospital cafeteria menu in figure 3A reflects standards that have been established by the menu planners. In order to meet the expectations of their customers, the planners establish these standards for the basic composition of the menu illustrated: luncheon entrees include a special hot sandwich and a plated hot entree; dinner entrees never include more than one extended or casserole item on the same day; only one starch is offered per meal; at least one green vegetable is offered every day; and like products are rotated. The menu is the basic standard that must be developed for the hospital cafeteria. It is the source of information regarding the need to establish specifications for items to be purchased, for recipes, and for standards for portions and services.

Why must standard purchase specifications be developed? The buyer needs them in order to know which items to solicit bids for. The purveyors need the standards so that they can fairly bid against one another for identical items that will satisfy the hospital's needs. The receiver must know the standards in order to check in each delivery properly, ascertain that the established standards have been met by the purveyors up to the time that the hospital assumes ownership of the food.

The precise information needed to establish the standard purchase specifications for all meat products required in the operation of a hospital cafeteria is contained in two readily available publications, *Meat Buyers Guide* by the National Association of Meat Purveyors and *Institutional Meat Purchase Specifications* by the U.S. Department of Agriculture. Another publication, *SPECS: The Comprehensive Food Service Purchasing & Specification Manual*, by R. B. Peddersen, includes an excellent section on meat purchasing and specifications as well as complete specifications for purchasing poultry, eggs, dairy products, fish, convenience foods, kosher food, produce, juices, jams and jellies, and miscellaneous groceries. (See the Bibliography for these titles.)

One page from a hospital cafeteria's meat specifications is illustrated in figure 3B. Similar information must be developed and utilized in the purchase of all categories of food items listed in the preceding paragraph. This task is not difficult, although it is time-consuming, and certainly it is educational if not actually enjoyable. The item on line 2 of figure 3B, *ground beef*, deserves particular notice. The figure indicates that the standard for that item is a U.S. Department of Agriculture grade of Good or Standard, MBG (*Meat Buyer's Guide*) item number 137, and IMPS (*Institutional Meat Purchase Specifications*) item number 137. It includes details that the ground beef be medium grind with a fat content of 20 to 22%. Were this specification not spelled out, any of four basic ground beef specifications with variable fat contents could be bid on, supplied, and used, resulting in unfair bid procedures and uncontrollable results.

Figure 3C illustrates a typical standard recipe and yield card. The exact weight and/or volume of each ingredient necessary to produce 115 5-oz portions of shrimp creole is given. The exact quantity given of each ingredient must be combined in the manner outlined to produce the yield standard and to meet the quality standard. There are many recipes in print for food items that could be served in a hospital cafeteria, and there are many variations of those recipes in the heads of the cooks who prepare them. In order to develop a standard recipe for each item served in the cafeteria, the food service administrator should read as many applicable recipes as possible, try the best ones, conduct taste tests comparing various recipes for the same item, and arrive at the best recipe for the item for use in the hospital cafeteria. Once the best recipe has been selected and extended to workable yields of desired portions, it becomes the standard for that food item. It is the standard that will be followed in purchasing food, it is the standard that the cooks must follow in production, it is the standard that the cafeteria will serve and will collect payment for, it is the standard that the customer will expect every time that item is ordered, and it is the standard that the hospital food service administrator will be ultimately responsible for.

Extending recipes to yield the most appropriate number of portions of the desired size is a simple mathematical procedure, given in many cookbooks. If the selected recipe for an item is available only in a format which produces 115 5-oz portions, the portion size can be adjusted by multiplying every ingredient by the desired portion size divided by the given portion size, for example:

Each ingredient x 4/5 = the given yield (115 portions)
in 4-oz portions

Each ingredient x 7/5 = the given yield (115 portions)
in 7-oz portions

The yield can be adjusted by multiplying each ingredient by the desired yield divided by the given yield, for example:

Each ingredient x 90/115 = 90 portions of the given size

Each ingredient x 180/115 = 180 portions of the given size

With the use of these simple formulas, selection of a standard recipe can be based on qualitative factors such as taste, texture, and appearance, and the necessary quantitative adjustments can be made independently of the qualitative decision.

The standards for portions and service result from menu standards, purchase standards, and recipe standards. A good way to provide quick reference to the portion and service standard is through a cafeteria portion and price book. A page from such a book is illustrated in figure 3D. Line 4 of figure 3D instructs the cafeteria server that the standard of service for shrimp creole is 5 oz served over 3 oz of rice. For this portion the cashier will charge $1.30. An additional tool that provides reference to the established service standard is a picture album containing photographs of each item on the serving line, illustrating the garnishment standard and pan presentation, and a plated portion of each item, illustrating the size of a portion as well as any accompaniments that may be part of the service standard, such as tartar sauce with fish, cranberry sauce with poultry, or pickles with a hamburger. Portion and service standards are, to a great degree, dictated by the makeup of the customers and the philosophy of the hospital toward cafeteria operation. Obtaining a proper return for the portion sizes and levels of service required in a particular hospital are discussed in chapter 5, Menu Pricing, and methods of ascertaining just what portions and services are most salable in the cafeteria are discussed in part B, Audit and Marketing Techniques.

Standards must be established to meet the legitimate demands placed on the hospital cafeteria. When an item such as shrimp creole appears on the menu, it must meet the standards of the menu planners as being from an appropriate food category—seafood, being in an appropriate form—casserole, being in an appropriate price range—$1.30, and being compatible with the accompanying and surrounding menu items. The purchase standards for the ingredients in the shrimp creole will demand such things as the shrimp being frozen, broken into pieces, peeled and deveined, and ready to cook. The recipe standard will place such demands on the food service worker as weighing exactly 12 lb of shrimp into each batch of 115 5-oz portions. The servers will serve a standard portion of 5 oz of shrimp creole on 3 oz of rice, and the cashier will charge exactly $1.30 for each such portion sold.

By all standards being established and met, the buyer knew what to buy, the purveyor knew what to bid on and deliver, the receiver knew what to accept, the cooks knew what to prepare and how to prepare it, the server knew what to serve and how to serve it, the cashier charged the correct price, the customers' demands of a $1.30 portion of shrimp creole were met, the predetermined gross profit was accomplished, and the food service administrator discharged his or her responsibility for a product that met all demands and expectations.

Figure 3A.
Hospital Cafeteria Menu

	Lunch	Dinner
Sunday, Dec. 16 Mulligatawny	Ham and Swiss Quiche Hot Roast Beef Sandwich Rissole Potatoes Squash Broccoli au Gratin	Sweet and Sour Pork on Rice Fried Chicken Buttered Rice Sliced Beets Cauliflower Polanaise
Monday, Dec. 17 Scotch Barley	Chicken a la King Baked Cheese Sandwich Whipped Sweet Potatoes Peas and Carrots Lima Beans	Baked Fish Chablis Ham Steak Buttered Noodles Green Beans Succotash
Tuesday, Dec. 18 New England Clam Chowder	Spaghetti and Meat Balls Hot Turkey Sandwich Baked Potato Mixed Vegetables Chopped Spinach	Omelet Lorraine Roast Beef Hash Brown Potatoes Garden Peas Stewed Tomatoes
Wednesday, Dec. 19 Chicken Noodle	Shrimp Creole on Rice Shaved Beef on a Hard Roll Buttered Rice Sliced Beets Creamed Corn	Roast Turkey and Dressing Beef Stew Whipped Potatoes Sliced Carrots Buttered Turnip Cubes
Thursday, Dec. 20 Minestrone	Baked Manicotti Grilled Ham and Cheese Sandwich Whipped Potatoes French Green Beans Buttered Broccoli	Fried Chicken Maryland Roast Pork Rissole Potatoes Creamed Spinach Buttered Cauliflower
Friday, Dec. 21 Tomato Rice	Macaroni and Cheese Monte Cristo Sandwich Baked Potato Beets l'Orange Succotash	Tacos Roast Beef Whipped Potatoes French Green Beans Red Cabbage
Saturday, Dec. 22 Corn Chowder	Fried Chicken Chili Dog Buttered Rice Wax Beans Chopped Spinach	Tuna Noodle Casserole Veal Parmesan Baked Potato Peas and Mushrooms Brussels Sprouts

Figure 3B.
Meat Specifications, Sample Page

No.	Item	Grade	MBG No.	IMPS No.	Details
	Beef				
1	Beef for stewing	Choice	135A	135A	Defatted. Seam fat ¼" max. at any point. 1" cubes, 20-22 per lb.
2	Ground beef	Good or Standard	137	137	Analytical fat content 20-22%. Medium grind.
3	Round, top, inside	Choice	168	168	14-17 lb boneless, split, tied or netted.
4	Round, bottom, outside	Choice	170	170	21-25 lb boneless, split, tied or netted.
5	Corned bottom round	Choice		606	"Selection #1" boneless. 25-28 lb, split and tied.
6A	Top sirloin butt	Choice	184	184	14-15 lb, split and tied. Boneless.
6B	Knuckle	Choice	167	167	14-15 lb, split. Boneless.
7	Flank steak	Choice	193	193	1¾-2 lb.
8	Chipped beef			619	Package 3 lb box.
9	Beef liver	US #1		703	4 oz portion—skinned, deveined, frozen.
10	Cubed steak	Choice	1101	1101	4 oz portion—frozen.
11	Ground beef patties	Good or Standard	1136	1136	4 oz portion—frozen, 20% maximum analytical fat.
12	Steak, sirloin strip, frozen	Choice	1180A	1180A	Individually wrapped. 9 oz boneless—extra short cut. 1" maximum flank edge from eye.
13	Steak, tenderloin, frozen	Choice	1189A	1189A	Individually wrapped. 7 oz defatted.
	Lamb				
1	Lamb patties	Choice or Good		1296A	3 oz portion—20-22% maximum analytical fat content. Frozen.
2	Lamb loin chops	Choice	1232	1232	6 oz portion. Film wrapped, frozen. Individually wrapped.
3	Lamb shanks			210	1-2 lb. For soup.

Figure 3C.
Standard Recipe and Yield Card

Category: Seafood
Item: Shrimp Creole

Portion: 5 oz on 3 oz rice

Ingredient	Yield	
	115 Servings	
Lemon juice	10	oz
Salt	2	oz
Vinegar	8	oz
Shrimp, broken P&D RTE	12	lb
Water	To cover	
Sauce tomatoes	3	#10 cans
Margarine	10	oz
Onions, sliced	3½	lb
Celery, sliced diagonally	4¾	lb
Green peppers, julienne	1¼	lb
Salt	1	oz
Oregano	⅔	oz
Thyme	⅓	oz
Cornstarch	10	oz

(front side)

Method:
1. Cook shrimp in lemon juice, salt, vinegar and water to cover. Simmer until cooked. Remove from heat.

2. Saute onions and celery in margarine. Add tomatoes, salt, oregano, thyme, and green peppers. Simmer until cooked.

3. Drain shrimp and add to sauce. Bring to boil and cook 5 minutes.

4. Mix cornstarch with liquid to form paste and add to mixture to thicken. Serve over 3 oz rice.

Utensils:
Can opener, scale, measuring cups and spoons, kettle, and knife.

(reverse side)

Figure 3D.
Portion and Price Book, Sample Page

Entree	Portion	Price	Comments
Baked fish	5 oz (raw)	$ 1.00	
Baked fish chablis	5 oz (raw)	1.00	W/1 oz sauce
Fried fish	5 oz (raw)	1.20	
Shrimp creole on rice	5 oz	1.30	Served on 3 oz rice
Seafood Newburg	5 oz	1.30	Served on 3 oz rice
Tuna noodle casserole	7 oz	1.00	
Fried shrimp	5 oz	2.00	W/1 oz cocktail sauce
Veal cutlet parmesan	3 oz	1.40	
Swiss veal crepe	1 ea	1.00	As portioned in kitchen
Baked ham	3 oz	1.00	
Ham steak	3 oz	1.10	W/3 oz fruit and sauce
Fresh ham	3 oz	1.10	W/#16 scoop of dressing
Cantonese sweet and sour pork	5 oz	1.20	On 3 oz rice

CHAPTER 4
DETERMINING FOOD COST

Standard food cost is obtained from costing out a standard recipe that lists ingredients, purchasing specifications, quantity, weight, portion size, and number of portions (see figure 4A).

STANDARD FOOD COST CALCULATION

The standard food cost calculation, as illustrated in figure 4A, is necessary for every item sold in a cafeteria. Most food service administrators know the unit food cost of a cup of coffee and a package of saltines because, in the case of coffee, it is so highly publicized and, in the case of saltines as well as many items that are resold as purchased, it is such a simple matter to divide the case price by the number of units in the case to find the unit food cost. However, the unit food cost for other items such as entrees, soups, desserts, and salads, as determined through use of the standard food cost recipe, is equally important in determining potential food cost and should not be avoided even though it is a laborious process to develop a complete file of costed recipes if none exists. Such a file is an indispensible tool to good food service management and, once developed, should be kept up to date to reflect current prices and actual recipe yield.

To obtain standard food costs for a recipe:
1. Multiply each recipe ingredient quantity by the ingredient cost per unit.
2. Total each ingredient cost.
3. Divide total recipe cost by the number of portions.
4. Add 6% of the food cost to cover incidental expenses such as shrinkage, catsup, salt, pepper, sugar, and so forth.

DEFINITIONS AND FORMULAS

In calculating food cost, the food service administrator can effectively utilize mathematical formulas in determining the amount to buy, portion costs, and the most economical product. The proper use of these mathematical formulas will improve the quality of decision making regarding food cost control.

As an aid in understanding these mathematical formulas, the following terms are defined:
- *As purchased (AP) weight* is the amount purchased, including bones, fat, unusable trim, outer layers, excess moisture, and so forth.

- *Edible portion (EP) weight* is the actual net amount obtained after processing has been performed.
- *Portion size* is the amount of food served to a customer.
- *Waste* is the amount of unusable food that is lost due to processing, cooking, and portioning. To determine the percentage of waste, divide the waste, or weight of the total loss, by AP weight of the product.

    Waste ÷ AP weight = waste %

- *Yield* is the amount of usable product remaining after all processing, cooking, and portioning is done. The yield figure is the reciprocal of percentage waste.

    Waste % + yield % = 100% AP weight

The *percentage of yield* can be obtained independently by dividing the AP weight into the net weight of the usable product.

    Yield ÷ AP weight = yield %

- *Portion factor* is the actual number of portions served per pound for any given product.

    16 oz ÷ portion size = portion factor

Note that several different portion factors for the same kind of product may be used in the same health care institution. A 3-oz and a 5-oz swiss steak may be used for patient and nonpatient meal service, respectively. Thus, each menu item has its own portion factor.

- *Portion divider* is the figure obtained by multiplying the portion factor by the percentage of yield of the product used.

    Yield % x portion factor = portion divider

EXAMPLE

The following example illustrates how these mathematical formulas can be applied in preparing a menu: The food service administrator has planned a roast beef menu for the hospital cafeteria to serve 200. The price of a top round of beef (raw) is $1.75 per pound, and the price of a precooked top round of beef is $2.20 per pound. The food service administrator wishes to determine (1) the amount of top round of beef to buy, (2) portion costs, and (3) which is the more economical product to buy, the raw or the precooked beef. Listed below are the mathematical formulas to be used in arriving at the best buy:

1. Determine the portion factor:

    16 oz ÷ 4 oz = 4 portion factor

2. Determine the portion divider:

    Yield % x portion factor = portion divider

    Item A: Top round of beef, raw: .50 x 4 = 2.0

Item B: Top round of beef, precooked: .85 x 4 = 3.4

3. Amount of top round of beef to buy:

Number of people ÷ portion divider = AP weight

Item A: 200 ÷ 2 = 100 lb

Item B: 200 ÷ 3.4 = 59 lb

4. Portion cost for the top round of beef:

AP price ÷ portion divider = portion cost

Item A: $1.75 ÷ 2.0 = $0.875

Item B: $2.20 ÷ 3.4 = $0.647

Obviously, the precooked top round of beef is the most economical product to purchase. But in the meat market, the price of one item in relation to a similar product often increases or decreases. At some stage of this fluctuation, it may become desirable to switch from one product to another to save money. Utilizing the portion divider, the food service administrator can readily determine this point of change as follows:

The portion cost for item A is obtained by dividing the portion divider (2.0) into the purchase price of $1.75. The portion cost for item A is $0.875.

Item A: AP price ÷ portion divider = portion cost

$1.75 ÷ 2.0 = $0.875

Now, to ascertain at what price to switch products, the portion cost of item A ($0.875) is multiplied by the portion divider of item B (3.4) to arrive at $2.975 per pound.

Item B: portion cost item A x portion divider item B = equal
market price

$0.875 x 3.4 = $2.975

The cost of $2.975 is the price at which both products are of equal value. However, if the purchase price of item B is below the equal value price of $2.975, then item B is a better buy. Consequently, when the price of item B is higher than the equal value price of $2.975, then item A is the better buy.

Figure 4A.
Standard Food Cost Calculation

___

Item: Chicken cacciatore
Yield: 48 servings
Portion: 1 cup

Method: Heat butter and saute garlic, onion, green peppers, and mushrooms for 5 minutes. Stir in sauce and white wine and herb blend. Simmer until thick and bubbly. Stir in poultry and reheat. Spoon sauce over cooked spaghetti and serve sprinkled with cheese.

Ingredient	Weight	Equivalent Measure	Cost
Butter or margarine	4 oz	½ cup	$ .09
Garlic, chopped	. . . .	6 cloves	.24
Onions, sliced	2 lb	1½ qt	.68
Green pepper, chopped	1 lb 8 oz	1½ qt	.60
Mushrooms, sliced	1 lb 8 oz	1½ qt	1.43
Marinara sauce	10 lb	1¼ gal	3.49
White wine	1 lb	1 pt	.74
Italian herb blend	. . . .	1 tbspn	.38
Poultry, diced, cooked	8 lb	1 gal	13.49
Spaghetti, cooked	8 lb	. . . .	.99
Parmesan cheese, grated	1 lb 8 oz	1½ qt	3.51
			25.64
For garnish, condiment and shrinkage (6%)			1.54
		Total cost	**$27.18**
		Cost per serving	**$ 0.566**

CHAPTER 5
MENU PRICING

The menu is one of several major marketing tools available to food service administrators. It identifies food items, the manner of preparation, and the price. It introduces the consumer to the cafeteria and establishes a certain mood. It also combines eye appeal, color, variety, contrast, and balance to merchandise the food, stimulate the appetite, and encourage consumers to return.

MENU AND MARKETING CONCEPTS

The price range and appeal of menu items are important determinants in attracting consumers. Menu prices certainly play an important part in determining what item to select.

Traditionally, a marketing strategy for a food service administrator consists of two distinct and yet interrelated areas, namely:
- *Target market*—a group of consumers to whom a cafeteria wishes to appeal, such as employees, physicians, students, and visitors.
- *Marketing mix*—a combination of food items and prices that appeals to consumers and makes the value attractive. Value as perceived by consumers may take many forms including convenience, fast service, pleasant atmosphere, trained personnel, clean environment, fair prices, and a nutritious menu.

The food service administrator needs to consider carefully competitors with similar menu and price structure, as well as the quality, cost, time, effort, and distance involved for consumers to prepare meals at home. In spite of the impact of market conditions on food and labor costs, menu prices must reflect the values and the current status of the cost structure of a cafeteria operation. However, if the food service administrator sets prices above a certain range, consumers will either trade down, eat at another establishment, or carry food with them.

CAFETERIA STANDARD COSTS

Cafeteria standard costs play an important role in determining the basis for menu pricing. The identification and clear definition of these standard costs of operation outline the scope and magnitude of cost behavior on menu pricing and the financial soundness of the cafeteria operation.

In addition to standard food cost discussed in chapter 4, cafeteria standard costs also cover the areas of labor, semifixed variable costs, fixed costs, and indirect costs. These costs are explained as follows:

1. *Standard labor cost.* Few food service administrators have determined labor cost per portion for each recipe. To allocate labor expenses, a time study can be developed to compute labor activities in these areas accurately:

    a. Pre-preparation of foods (washing, cutting, trimming, slicing, and so forth)

    b. Assembly of ingredients (weighing, mixing, blending, forming, and so forth)

    c. Preparation of foods (roasting, baking, frying, and so forth)

    d. Portioning of foods

    e. Delay time (waiting, watching, breaks, and so forth)

    f. Cleanup time

    Total time and labor cost (including fringe benefits) can then be determined for each recipe. It is appropriate to determine the cost of a standard portion based on the number of portions normally produced at one time.

2. *Semivariable costs.* Semivariable costs are those costs that are composed of one part that is independent of volume and one part that varies proportionately with volume, such as supplies, travel, telephone, labor, repairs, and improvements. These costs are also called controllable costs.

3. *Fixed costs.* Fixed costs are those that are unresponsive to changes in volume, such as depreciation and insurance. These costs are commonly known as uncontrollable expenses.

4. *Indirect costs.* Indirect costs are expenses generated by other departments of the health care institution in the course of providing a general service to all departments. These indirect costs may include expenses for administrative and general costs, building depreciation, heat, light and power costs, debt costs, and service departments such as personnel, accounting, housekeeping, and payroll.

The food service administrator can determine from current cafeteria operating statements and/or from the accounting office what percentage of cafeteria sales is attributed to semivariable costs, fixed costs, and indirect costs. It is suggested that the ratio of these expenses to sales be calculated on an annual basis and adjusted whenever the need arises.

SALES MIX

The food service administrator uses the sales mix approach to analyze in depth the impact of individual menu items on each other and on the aggregate. This review shows how menu items in a specific food group compete with each other for customer selection. Sales mix details the selling price of each menu item, the unit food cost, the cost of food, the number of servings sold, the sales mix percentages, the total sales, the total food cost, the contribution to other costs, and the percentage of contribution to other costs.

Figure 5A shows an analysis of the sales mix of a daily menu in a cafeteria. The information presented in figure 5A is fairly simple to obtain. Column 1,

"Menu," and column 2, "Selling Price," are given in the cafeteria's price book and are posted on the menu board. Column 3, "Unit Food," is found on the food cost recipe card (figure 4A). Column 4, "Food Cost %," is determined by dividing column 3 by column 2 and multiplying by 100, for example:

Fillet of cod: $(.80 \div 1.75) \times 100 = 46\%$

Column 5, "Number Sold," can be found in the records kept for that day's menu. The number of portions sold of each item should appear on the production record for the meal, on the cafeteria hot entree requisition, and on the readout of the electronic cash register in those cafeterias that have that piece of equipment.

The data can be retrieved from manually kept records such as a Daily Production Record (see figure 5B). The production staff can use this form to record issues from which returns are subtracted to arrive at the number used of each item. The cafeteria staff can use it to record receipts from which leftovers are subtracted to arrive at the number sold of each item. Variations of the form, with appropriate items listed, can also be used in cold food areas. Most important, as long as the number of servings sold of each item has been accurately recorded, the food service administrator can use these forms to determine the consumption of each food item produced and sold. The usage of those items that do not pass through a production process prior to sale can be determined by reviewing the cafeteria requisition for the item (see figure 5C, Resale Food Requisition).

Column 6 in figure 5A, "Sales Mix %," is found by dividing the number of portions sold of an individual item by the total portions sold of all items and multiplying by 100, for example:

Fillet of cod: $(162 \div 799) \times 100 = 21\%$

Column 7, "Total Sales," is the selling price multiplied by the number sold. Column 8, "Total Food Cost," is the unit food cost multiplied by the number sold.

Column 9, "Contribution to Other Costs," is total sales minus total food cost. Column 10, "% Contribution to Other Costs," is the individual item's contribution divided by the total contribution and multiplied by 100, for example:

Fillet of cod: $(153.90 \div 606.81) \times 100 = 25\%$

Figure 5A, Sales Mix of a Daily Menu, compares the sales of five entree items, the food cost, and the amount contributed to other costs. The sale of fillet of cod, hamburger, and chicken with dressing represented 79% of sales (column 6) and contributed 81% to other costs (column 10). The distribution of sales among these three entree items ranges from 21% to 30% whereas the remaining menu items, lasagna and super dog, together represented only 21% of sales and contribute 18% to other costs. The food service administrator now has this information available to make valuable decisions affecting the production and service of food. The question arises, should the super dog be dropped? Perhaps the price of 85 cents for a super dog may have taken sales away from other high-priced menu items. Moreover, a case can be made that there is no need to feature hamburger and super dogs on the same menu.

Now, what about the lasagna? Should lasagna be on the menu? The preparation of lasagna takes labor, the cost of the ingredients is high, and trained cooks are needed to prepare it. But how often is lasagna prepared at home? Consumers may prefer not to prepare it at home but to purchase it when eating away from home.

These alternatives would require careful study by the food service administrator, because the impact of any decision regarding these choices of entree items will affect the consumer as well as the food service staff and sales.

EFFECT OF SALES VOLUME ON PROFIT MARGIN

When serious attempts are made to expand the contribution of profit margin to defray other costs, the food service administrator should consider the concepts of added value to menu items and differential pricing structure. Examples of the use of these concepts follow.

Certainly no food service administrator can afford to ignore the large, growing and profitable soft drink, coffee, and ice cream markets. According to a 1978 survey, 29% of all beverages ordered away from home were soft drinks (ref. 1). Contrary to general belief, coffee came in second with 19% and all other beverages had percentages far below this figure. Actually, soft drinks carry a higher profit margin than other beverages. A typical soft drink has a food cost of between 17% to 19% but coffee carries a 35% food cost. In fact, the penny profit from soft drinks often exceeds the profit from coffee by more than 60%.

To take advantage of the simple but effective merchandising technique of added value, the food service administrator first must review the price levels of soft drinks. This price evaluation can be accomplished by analyzing the market situation and also by working with the national soft drink manufacturers. The soft drink suppliers have the expertise and the necessary research to aid in developing a plan to maximize profits.

In the majority of cases, an adjustment in the ratio of price to size mix will generate greater profits than an across-the-board price increase. Of course, the sizing of soft drinks will vary somewhat depending on the region, the weather, and the cafeteria environment. However, the ideal cup mix is a three-size combination of 8 oz, 12 oz and 16 oz. When properly priced, this size mix will meet consumer needs while maximizing soft drink profits.

An important principle to follow when pricing different-sized soft drinks is value pricing, which suggests that consumers should get more for their money as the size of the drink increases. For example, a 12-oz cup priced at 30 cents offers the product at 2.5 cents per ounce. But the large 16-oz size priced at 36 cents is 2.25 cents per ounce, thus providing consumers with a positive incentive (discount) to trade up to the larger, more profitable size. In addition, there is no increase in labor costs no matter what size is sold, but there is a greater profit contribution to costs by selling the larger size.

Another area of soft drink merchandising that deserves more attention is the icing of soft drinks. Icing directly affects the taste, appeal, and salability of a drink. The result of over-icing contributes to poor quality soft drinks through accelerated dilution, which causes drinks to be weak and flat and to lose their distinctive flavor.

Moreover, the amount of ice in a soft drink also has a psychological affect on the consumer. A consumer who finishes a drink and finds a lot of ice left in the glass will feel cheated and will have a poor price-value perception. There should be just a trace of ice left after consumption so that the consumer has a high perception of the value and quality of the drink. Ice is an important element in the consumer's enjoyment of a soft drink. Research has shown the optimum amount of ice to put in a glass is one-third of the container height.

The sale of soft ice cream provides another example of increasing the profit margin. Again, a national manufacturer of soft ice cream is in a position to provide expertise in merchandising soft ice cream at a higher profit margin. Specifically, suppliers of soft ice cream can assist in establishing operating standards for overruns, size of dish or cone, and merchandising and pricing techniques. An example of how to price soft ice cream portions profitably follows:

1. Determine total cost per portion. Add up costs for ounces of product served plus topping, container, spoon, and so forth. Cost charts that provide many of these costs quickly are readily available from national vendors. For example, a 7-oz soft-serve sundae has the following costs:

    $ .1264 7 oz soft-serve @ $2.60/gal
    .0504 1 oz syrup @ $5.80/gal
    .0344 1 oz whipped creme @ $1.10/qt
    .0107 one whole cherry @ $7.50/gal
    .0233 cup
    .0083 spoon
    ─────────
    $0.2535 Total cost

2. Determine what percentage of the selling price the total cost per portion should be. In this example, the food service administrator wants the cost per portion to be 33.3% of the selling price.

3. Determine the selling price by dividing the total cost per portion ($0.2535) by the desired percentage that the cost per portion will be of the selling price (33%).

    $0.2535 ÷ 33.3% = $0.7613

Thus the selling price of a 7-oz soft-serve sundae is 76 cents, to realize a 66.7% gross profit.

Another popular approach to maximizing the contribution to indirect costs is the addition to the "Today's Special" item of a complimentary item with a differential pricing structure. This added value enhances the menu and offers the consumer a good selection at a good value. To illustrate the concept of added value to "Today's Special," the menu offerings Burger and Super Dog listed in figure 5A are modified in figure 5D, Sales Mix of a Daily Menu with Added Value, as follows:

Burger with french fries and dispensed beverage at $1.65
Super Dog with french fries and dispensed beverage at $1.45

This particular merchandising approach promotes the sale of a complete sandwich purchase at an attractive price. This technique builds on such national advertising by fast-food chains as "Hamburger, French Fries, Large

Coke for 99 Cents." The familiarity of this type of advertising encourages more sales and contributes more profitability. The selling price of "Today's Special" may be discounted by 5 or 10 cents from *a la carte* prices to promote the consumer's perception of good value. The odd-cent pricing of 99 cents, $1.69, or $1.99 also has a positive psychological effect on the purchaser.

IMPACT OF MENU CHANGES ON PROFITABILITY

Price changes resulting from menu changes can be seen by comparing figures 5A and 5D. The result of added value on two menu items has increased the average check from $1.30 to $1.52, increased the amount of contribution to other costs by $127.16, or 21%, and decreased the average cost of food from 40% to 38%.

With the use of this simple technique, the food service administrator can increase cafeteria sales, lower the ratio of food cost to sales, and improve the profit margin with the same labor costs. As an illustration of the scope and magnitude of this impact on the profitability of the cafeteria, the price range and the amount of contribution realized toward paying for other operating costs are outlined in figure 5E, Price Range and Contribution to Other Costs.

DETERMINANTS AND RESTRICTIONS IN PRICING A MENU

Buchanan (ref. 2) has outlined these important strategies in pricing a menu:
- Consumers should be offered good value for their money
- The menu, service, and atmosphere should be developed to meet consumer's needs, preferences, and attitudes
- The basics of menu pricing depend on a well developed budget
- Low-priced menu items should provide the maximum contribution toward paying for all costs
- Menu items that are priced too high may reduce sales and increase operating costs
- Menu prices should be raised to correspond with advertised increases in newspapers or with published government reports or surveys; the price of a particular menu item should be increased when the cost of that item increases substantially
- Uniqueness of the product and creative promotion or merchandising require a higher price
- Menu items with high cost or with high risk of spoilage require a higher price
- Menu items with low cost or with low risk of spoilage require a lower price
- Volume is increased through marketing research, promotion, merchandising, and personal service
- Analysis of sales mix and adequate financial records, including food, labor, supplies and other costs, are indispensable to proper pricing
- Odd-cent pricing, ethnic foods, and offering menu items in combination provide a definite attraction
- Pricing decisions must be based on market factors of the competitive

conditions, prices of food in supermarkets, consumer demand, price relationships, and the determination of the full cost of each unit of service

- Excessive price spread among entrees encourages consumers to order lower-priced items; if the most expensive entree is more than two times the price of the least expensive item or if there is a definite concentration of entree selection among the less expensive items, excessive price spread probably exists
- Menu price should be planned to provide consumers with the perception of receiving good value for their money. Sales volume increases through the consumer's satisfaction and perception of value
- Loss leaders may be used, from time to time, to draw consumers into the cafeteria
- Menu prices should be evaluated frequently
- There should be no charge for small items
- Consumers expect to pay certain prices for specific items
- Menu prices are frequently maintained at the same level regardless of the prices in the market place
- Consumers will not pay above a perceived maximum price for an item
- Consumers will not pay for menu items that are far above a competitor's range

APPROACHES TO MENU PRICING SYSTEMS

The old rule "To figure the selling price of a menu item, multiply food cost by a factor of 2½ to obtain a 40% food cost" is not an appropriate method for pricing food items. This method of menu pricing tends to set the selling price of low food cost and high labor-intensive items too low and to set the selling price of high food cost and low labor menu items too high. For example, consider these two menu items priced by this method:

	Beef Stew	New York Strip Steak, 10 oz
Food cost	$1.21	$3.36
Selling price at 2½ factor:	$3.05	$8.40

It is obvious that this method of menu pricing is not based on an estimate of the labor cost required in the preparaton of the beef stew or the New York strip steak. A second weakness of this menu pricing method is the large spread in the selling prices between those two food items. To price a cafeteria menu item correctly, the food service administrator must take into account expenses for food; labor and employee benefits; supplies; wear and tear on the equipment, furniture, and facility; and costs associated with production, merchandising, and sales. In addition, the food service administrator needs to consider the financial objectives of the institution, the competition, the supply market, the environment, and the perceived value of the food and service to the customer. As an example of operating costs that should be included in menu pricing, see figures 5F, Cafeteria Operating Statement, and 5G, Financial Indicators.

Three menu pricing approaches that meet appropriate menu pricing objectives are described below. This menu pricing presentation centers on methods and concepts only; the examples are not intended to support the operational ratios, dollar figures, or costs given.

PRIME COST PRICING SYSTEM

The prime cost pricing method is based on adding food cost to labor cost and dividing the sum by the prime cost ratio, that is, the sum of the ratios of food and labor costs to total direct expenses. Thus, the general formula for menu pricing under the prime cost pricing approach is as follows:

$$\text{Selling price} = \frac{\$ \text{ food cost} + \$ \text{ labor cost}}{\text{prime cost ratio}}$$

To compute the food cost, labor cost, and the prime cost ratio, refer to figures 5F and 5G. The value of meal equivalent is $3.00 (figure 5G) and the ratios for food and labor costs are 42% and 38% respectively. These ratios are taken from figure 5F, "Year to date-Actual" column. The value and the breakdown of the various components of meal equivalent are outlined in figure 5H, Value of Meal Equivalent. The labor cost for the meat item is 46 cents. Now apply this information to the previous examples of the beef stew and the New York strip steak, and calculate the selling price as follows:

Beef stew:

$$\text{Selling price} = \frac{\$1.21 \text{ food cost} + \$0.46 \text{ labor cost} = \$1.67}{42\% + 38\% = 80\%}$$

Selling price = $2.09

New York strip steak:

$$\text{Selling price} = \frac{\$3.36 \text{ food cost} + \$0.46 \text{ labor cost} = \$3.82}{42\% + 38\% = 80\%}$$

Selling price = $4.78

The result of this method of menu pricing is to decrease the menu selling prices of the beef stew and the New York strip steak and to narrow the price spread to a tolerable level.

If the prime cost ratio is changed from 80% to 50%, the impact of this change is illustrated as follows:

Beef stew:

$$\text{Selling price} = \frac{\$1.21 \text{ food cost} + \$0.46 \text{ labor cost} = \$1.67}{42\% + 38\% = 50\%}$$

Selling price = $3.34

New York strip steak:

$$\text{Selling price} = \frac{\$3.36 \text{ food cost} + \$0.46 \text{ labor cost} = \$3.82}{42\% + 38\% = 50\%}$$

Selling price = $7.64

The effect of the prime cost method when compared to the 2½ pricing factor method is to increase the selling price of the low food cost and high labor-intensive items (beef stew) and to lower the selling price of the high food cost and low labor items (New York strip steak). Also, it decreases the large spread in the selling prices between two or more items. When these simple examples are expanded to a typical food service cafeteria menu featuring appetizers, entrees, desserts, and beverages, with separate lunch and dinner menus, the selling price calculation can become more cumbersome. To meet this challenge, these tables are provided to highlight the basic information required in the computation of a complete cafeteria menu:

1. Figure 5H, Value of Meal Equivalent, outlines the average selling price for meat, potato, vegetable, salad, dessert, beverage, and the total value of a meal. The percentage column assigns a weighted rating to each meal component based on the total value of the meal equivalent. This information is helpful in the assignment of cost for labor, food, supplies, other expenses, and indirect expenses. The labor cost for a meal equivalent was calculated from information contained in figures 5F and 5G. For example, in figure 5F, the actual cost of labor, in the "Year to date-Actual" column, is $284,014, and the number of meal equivalents in figure 5G is 248,864. $284,014 divided by 248,864 is $1.14, the labor cost per meal equivalent in figure 5H. The same calculations were made for other operating costs per meal equivalent and are recorded in figure 5H under the appropriate columns.

2. Another method of effectively pricing a hospital cafeteria menu requires the capturing of the total number of menu items prepared for both patient and nonpatient activities and calculating the number of labor hours involved in the production and service of food for each activity. The production and service hours may include supervision, forecasting, purchasing, receiving, storage, food preparation, cooking, baking, grilling, sanitation, and serving personnel for nonpatient areas. Figure 5I, Labor Cost Based on Menu Items, details the procedure for calculating the labor cost per menu item. Column 1 lists the menu items offered in the food service department. Column 2 shows the number of menu items prepared and handled in a central location for patient and nonpatient activities. Column 3 assigns a relative value unit (RVU) for each menu item based on the amount of effort required to prepare and assemble these items. Column 4 distributes the total production hours based on the RVU and assigns each menu item with the appropriate labor hours for patient and nonpatient activities. Column 5 lists the total of nonpatient service labor hours and assigns service labor hours based on RVU. Column 6 is the total of nonpatient labor hours as shown in columns 4 and 5. Column 7 distributes the total nonpatient labor minutes per menu item. Column 8 calculates the nonpatient labor cost at $6.25 per hour for each menu item. For example, on the average, the labor cost to prepare and serve an entree in a nonpatient area is 65 cents. This figure may assist the food service administrator in properly ascertaining the labor cost per individual menu item.

3. Figure 5J, Value and Cost Analysis of Meal Equivalent, summarizes the operating costs for a meal and coordinates the operating cost percen-

tages with the cafeteria operating statement as shown in figure 5F.

4. Figure 5K, Costs and Ratios Analysis of Meal Equivalent, illustrates the relationship between the individual components of meal costs and ratios.

The information contained in figures 5J and 5K on operating cost percentages (Labor, Food, Supply, Other Expenses, and Contribution to Indirect Cost) can be successfully used as a basis for pricing the menu items. Indeed, the availability of this information will enable the food service administrator to lay the foundation for a detailed and objective menu pricing.

In summary, Patterson (ref. 3) ascribed these advantages for using the prime costing approach:

- It is a system that makes sure that the more expensive items are priced to produce the greatest dollar profit.
- By using a standard labor cost factor for all items in a given menu class (such as entrees), price spread is reduced from what it would be if only food cost were considered. The reduced price spread is a factor that encourages consumers to order the higher priced and more profitable items.
- By allocating labor costs to menu items and considering them along with food costs, some control over the two largest cost segments on a profit-and-loss statement is achieved.

MODIFICATION TO THE PRIME COST PRICING SYSTEM

According to Buchanan (ref. 4), in the Modified Prime Cost Pricing System the food cost is multiplied by a labor factor representing the degree of effort (low-, medium-, and high-skilled labor) required in the preparation of a product. The formula is:

Food cost x labor factor = selling price

The degree of effort is based on the following factors:
- The degree of labor convenience built into the purchased food product
- The type of labor rate involved in handling and preparaton of the menu time

To a large extent, the assignment of labor cost for the preparation of menu items at varying degrees of product convenience is a subjective determination. However, to simplify the labor cost calculation, Buchanan developed a matrix, Labor Factor Guide. The matrix details the degree of product convenience from high to average to low on the horizontal axis and coordinates it with the labor rate of low, average, and high on the vertical axis. A matrix for a cafeteria may be developed in a similar fashion (see figure 5L).

For example, to compute the selling price of beef stew and New York strip steak, suppose that the labor factor is high (3) for beef stew, as a task identified in square 9 (Casseroles), and the labor factor is low (2.25) for New York strip steak, as a task identified in square 1 (Sliced Meats). Then the calculation will be as follows:

Beef stew selling price = $1.21 x 3 = $3.63

New York strip steak selling price = $3.36 x 2.25 = $7.56

It should be noted that each cafeteria operation has its unique menu characteristics, level of skilled labor, and availability of products on the market. Thus, each food service administrator has to develop a labor factor matrix based on the actual characteristics of the menu, recipes, labor market, environment, and the institution. Of course, the development of this matrix is subjective in nature, but the ultimate moderating factor for the determination of menu pricing will be the competition, the reaction of the customers, and the attainment of the financial objective of the cafeteria and the institution.

COST-PLUS-PROFIT PRICING SYSTEM

Jack Welsh, now professor emeritus of food science and nutrition, University of Missouri at Columbia, advanced a menu pricing concept that included the cost of food ingredients, direct labor and benefits, other operating expenses, fixed expenses, and profit. The basic formula is as follows:

Food ingredient cost + labor and benefit costs + controllable cost + fixed cost + profit = 100% = selling price

To calculate the selling price of beef stew, the food ingredient cost amounts to $1.21; figure 5H, Value of Meal Equivalent, shows labor cost at 46 cents, and Figure 5F, Cafeteria Operating Statement, "Year to date-Actual" column reflects supply expenses at 7%, other expenses at 1%, and required contribution to indirect expenses at 12%. The cost-plus-profit pricing equation is solved in this manner:

$1.21 + $0.46 + 7% + 1% + 12% = 100% = selling price
$1.21 + $0.46 = 100% - (7% + 1% + 12%)
$1.67 = 80%
$1.67 ÷ .80 = 100% = $2.09

Thus, $2.09 is the recommended selling price to produce a 12% contribution to indirect expenses.

Similarly, to calculate the selling price of New York strip steak, the cost of the New York strip steak is $3.36, figure 5H shows labor cost at 46 cents, and figure 5F indicates that supply, other expenses, and required contribution to indirect expenses are 7%, 1% and 12% respectively. The selling price is computed in this manner:

$3.36 + $0.46 + 7% + 1% + 12% = 100% = selling price
$3.36 + $0.46 = 100% - (7% + 1% + 12%)
$3.82 = 80%
$3.82 ÷ .80 = 100% = $4.78

In summary, it should be noted that all these menu cost pricing systems have merits. However, food service administrators need to analyze them carefully, adopt the method appropriate to their own operation, and check their own pricing strategy against each method to insure that the system they use is fair, simple, and valid and is meeting the institution's financial objectives for the cafeteria operation.

Figure 5A.
Sales Mix of a Daily Menu

1	2	3	4	5	6	7	8	9	10
Menu Item	Selling price, $	Unit food cost, $	Food cost, %	Number sold	Sales mix, %	Total sales, $	Total food costs, $	Contribution to other costs, $	Contribution to other costs, %
Fillet of cod	1.75	.80	46	162	21	283.50	129.90	153.90	25
Burger	1.05	.38	36	217	28	227.85	82.46	145.39	24
Chicken w/dressing	1.35	.52	38	232	30	313.20	120.64	192.56	32
Lasagna	1.30	.50	38	96	12	124.80	48.00	76.80	13
Super dog	.85	.32	38	72	09	61.20	23.04	38.16	6
Total				**779**	**100**	**1,010.55**	**403.74**	**606.81**	**100**

$$\text{Average food cost, \%} = \frac{\text{Total food cost}}{\text{Total sales}} \quad \text{or} \quad \frac{\$\ 403.74}{\$1,010.55} = 40\%$$

$$\text{Average contribution to other costs, \%} = \frac{\text{Total contribution to other costs}}{\text{Total sales}} \quad \text{or} \quad \frac{\$\ 606.81}{\$1,010.55} = 60\%$$

$$\text{Average check, \$} = \frac{\text{Total sales}}{\text{Total servings sold}} \quad \text{or} \quad \frac{\$1,010.55}{779} = \$1.30$$

Figure 5B.
Daily Production Record

DAY_____   DATE_____

Menu Item	Unit/ Portion	Ordered	Issued or Rec'd	Leftover	Used
Lunch					
Cream of mushroom soup	Gal				
Beef burgundy	5-oz				
Grilled Reuben sandwich	Each				
Noodles	3-oz				
Peas and onions	3-oz				
Wax beans	3-oz				
Dinner					
Cream of mushroom soup	Gal				
Seafood Newburg	5-oz				
Chicken Hawaiian	1/4				
Rice	3-oz				
Buttered carrots	3-oz				
Broccoli au gratin	3-oz				

Figure 5C.
Resale Food Requisition

Day_____ Date_____ Ordered_____ Delivered_____ Received_____

Item	Unit/ Portion	Par	Inventory	Order	Delivered	Unit Price	Cost
Apples	Ea	12					
Oranges	Ea	12					
Bananas	Ea	12					
Sherbet, orange	4-oz cup	24					
Sherbet, raspberry	4-oz cup	24					
Ice cream bars	Ea	24					
Ice cream sandwiches	Ea	30					
Ice cream cup, chocolate	4-oz cup	36					
Ice cream cup, vanilla	4-oz cup	36					
Milk, homogenized	½ pt	48					
Milk, skim	½ pt	48					
Milk, chocolate	½ pt	24					
Yogurt, vanilla	8-oz	6					
Yogurt, plain	8-oz	3					
Yogurt, assorted flavors	8-oz	12					
Juice, apple	4-oz ind.	24					
Juice, cranberry	4-oz ind.	24					
Juice, grape	4-oz ind.	24					
Juice, grapefruit	4-oz ind.	24					
Juice, orange	4-oz ind.	48					

Figure 5D.
Sales Mix of a Daily Menu with Added Value

Menu	Selling price, $	Unit food cost, $	Food cost, %	Number sold	Sales mix, %	Total sales, $	Total food costs, $	Contribution to other costs, $	Contribution to other costs, %
Fillet of cod	1.75	.80	46	162	21	283.50	129.60	153.90	21
Burger w/fries and beverage	1.65	.54	33	217	28	358.05	117.18	240.87	33
Chicken w/dressing	1.35	.52	30	232	30	313.20	120.64	192.56	26
Lasagna	1.30	.50	38	96	12	124.80	48.00	76.80	11
Super dog w/fries and beverage	1.45	.48	33	72	9	104.40	34.56	69.84	9
Total				779	100	1,183.95	449.98	733.97	100

Average food cost, % = $\dfrac{\text{Total food cost}}{\text{Total sales}}$ or $\dfrac{\$\ 449.98}{\$1,183.95}$ = 38%

Average contribution to other costs, % = $\dfrac{\text{Total contribution to other costs}}{\text{Total sales}}$ or $\dfrac{\$\ 733.97}{\$1,183.95}$ = 62%

Average check, $ = $\dfrac{\text{Total sales}}{\text{Total servings sold}}$ or $\dfrac{\$1,183.95}{779}$ = $1.52

Figure 5E.
Price Range and Contribution to Other Costs

Menu item	Price, $	Contribution to other costs, $	Contribution to other costs with value added, $
Fillet of cod	1.75	153.90	153.90
Burger	1.05	145.39	
Burger w/value added	1.65		240.87
Super dog	.85	38.16	
Super dog w/value added	1.45		69.84
Chicken w/dressing	1.35	192.56	192.56
Lasagna	1.30	76.80	76.80
		606.81	**733.97**

Figure 5F.
Cafeteria Operating Statement, XYZ Hospital

	Current Period: January				Year to Date: July-January			
	Actual	**Budget**	**Variance**	**% Variance**	**Actual**	**Budget**	**Variance**	**% Variance**
Cafeteria sales (100%)	$102,423	$ 94,500	($7,923)	8.4	$746,592	$661,500	($85,092)	12.9
Salaries and Benefits								
Salaries	32,764	32,018	(746)	(2.3)	243,120	226,210	(16,910)	(7.5)
Fringe benefits	6,878	7,039	161	2.3	40,894	49,076	8,182	18.8
Total Salaries and Benefits	39,642 (39%)	39,057 (41%)	(585)	(1.5)	284,014 (38%)	275,286 (41%)	(8,728)	(3.2)
Food Expenses								
Meat, fish, poultry	20,036	18,654	(1,382)	(7.4)	147,402	127,802	(19,600)	(15.3)
Fresh produce	685	631	(54)	(8.6)	5,778	5,557	221	(3.9)
Frozen vegetable	1,273	1,350	77	5.7	10,557	11,113	556	5.0
Canned goods	15,697	13,891	(1,806)	(13.0)	108,730	94,462	(14,268)	(15.0)
Milk	2,539	2,778	239	8.6	23,614	22,226	(1,388)	(6.2)
Bakery	1,763	2,386	623	26.0	17,835	16,670	(1,165)	(7.0)
Total Food Expenses	41,993 (41%)	39,690 (42%)	(2,303)	(5.8)	313,916 (42%)	277,830 (42%)	(36,086)	(13.0)
Supply Expenses								
Disposal	4,160	3,656	(504)	(13.8)	28,177	24,647	(3,530)	(14.0)
Cleaning supplies	1,107	1,016	(91)	(8.96)	6,121	5,021	(1,100)	(21.9)
China and silverware	1,740	1,943	203	10.3	15,225	15,975	750	4.69
Total Supply Expenses	7,007 (7%)	6,615 (7%)	392	(5.9)	49,523 (7%)	45,643 (7%)	(3,880)	(8.5)
Other Expenses								
Depreciation	241	197	(44)	(22.3)	1,537	1,451	86	(5.9)
Laundry	169	180	11	6.1	1,143	975	168	(17.0)
Miscellaneous expenses	237	18	(219)	(1,216.6)	622	560	62	(11.0)
Office supplies	69	84	15	17.8	469	385	84	(21.8)
Rental equipment	153	196	43	22.3	3,877	3,594	283	(7.9)
Repairs	461	215	(246)	(114.4)	2,682	2,560	122	(4.8)
Telephone	51	55	4	7.3	168	150	18	(12.0)
Total Other Expenses	1,381 (1%)	945 (1%)	(436)	(46.1)	10,498 (1%)	9,675 (2%)	823	(8.5)
Total Direct Expenses	90,023 (88%)	86,307 (91%)	(3,716)	4.3	657,951 (88%)	608,434 (92%)	(49,517)	(8.1)
Contribution to Indirect Expenses	12,400 (12%)	8,193 (9%)	(4,207)	51.3	88,641 (12%)	53,066 (8%)	(35,575)	(67.0)

Figure 5G.
Financial Indicators

Current Period: January		Year to date: July-Jan.	
$	0.85	Sales/customer	$	0.85
	3.00	Value/meal equivalent		3.00
	4.94	Meal equivalent/paid hour		5.03
	855.00	Meal equivalent/FTE		6,089.00
	3,020.00	Customer/FTE		21,402.00
	2,566.00	Sales/FTE		18,267.00
$	310.62	Sales less direct expense/FTE	$	2,169.00
	120,576	Customer count		874,716
	34,141	Meal equivalent		248,864
	6,906	Paid hours		49,500
	39.92	FTE		40.87

Figure 5H.
Value of Meal Equivalent

	Average selling price, $	Per-centage	Total labor cost, $	Total food cost, $	Total supply cost, $	Total other expenses, $	Total direct expenses, $	Contribution to indirect expenses, $
Meat	1.20	40	0.46	0.50	.08	0.02	1.06	.14
Potato	.30	10	.12	.12	.02	.01	.27	.04
Vegetable	.30	10	.11	.13	.02	.01	.27	.04
Salad	.45	15	.17	.19	.03		.39	.05
Dessert	.45	15	.17	.19	.03		.39	.05
Beverage	.30	10	.11	.13	.02		.26	.04
Total value/meal equivalent	3.00	100	1.14	1.26	0.02	0.04	2.64	.36

Figure 5I.
Labor Cost Based on Menu Items

1	2			3	4			5	6	7	8
	Number of Items Prepared			Relative Value Unit	Production Labor Hours			Nonpatient Service Labor, Hrs	Total Nonpatient Labor, Hrs	Total Nonpatient Labor, Min/Unit	Nonpatient Labor Cost/Unit at $6.25/Hr
Menu Item	Patient	Nonpatient	Total*		Patient	Nonpatient	Total*				
Entree	4,673	5,946	10,619	3.00	158	200	358	416	616	6.2	.65
Vegetable	3,761	1,880	5,641	.75	59	30	89	104	134	4.3	.45
Soup	1,996	897	2,893	.50	41	19	60	69	88	5.9	.61
Salad	3,721	4,906	8,177	1.50	72	107	179	208	315	3.8	.40
Dessert	6,897	3,099	9,996	.75	61	28	89	104	132	2.5	.26
Sandwich	907	3,217	4,124	1.25	33	116	149	173	289	5.4	.56
Beverage	10,999	23,373	34,372	.25	10	20	30	35	55	.14	.01
Total	32,504	43,318	75,822	8.00	434	520	954	1,109	1,629		
Percentage	43%	57%	100%		45%	55%	100%				

*Data are based on a seven-day-per-week activity.

Figure 5J.
Value and Cost Analysis of Meal Equivalent

Value of Meal Equivalent	$3.00	Percentage, 100%
Labor cost	1.14	38
Food cost	1.26	42
Supply cost	.20	7
Other expenses	.04	1
Total direct expenses	2.64	88
Contribution/indirect expenses	.36	12

Figure 5K.
Costs and Ratios Analysis of Meal Equivalent

	Meat	Potato	Vegetable	Salad	Dessert	Beverage	Total
Average selling price	$1.20	$0.30	$0.30	$0.45	$0.45	$0.30	$3.00
Labor, cost	$0.46	$0.12	$0.11	$0.17	$0.17	$0.11	$1.14
Labor, %	38%	40%	37%	37%	37%	37%	38%
Food, cost	$0.50	$0.12	$0.13	$0.19	$0.19	$0.13	$1.26
Food, %	42%	40%	43%	42%	42%	43%	42%
Supply, cost	$0.08	$0.02	$0.02	$0.03	$0.03	$0.02	$0.20
Supply, %	6%	6%	6%	6%	6%	6%	6%
Other expenses, cost	$0.02	$0.01	$0.01	—	—	—	$0.04
Other expenses, %	2%	3%	3%	—	—	—	1%
Total direct expenses, cost	$1.06	$0.27	$0.27	$0.39	$0.39	$0.26	$2.64
Total direct expenses, %	88%	90%	90%	90%	90%	90%	88%
Contribution/direct expenses, cost	$0.14	$0.04	$0.04	$0.05	$0.05	$0.04	$0.36
Contribution/direct expenses, %	12%	13%	13%	11%	11%	14%	12%

Figure 5L.
Labor Factor Guide

Degree of Product Convenience

	High	Average	Low
Low	1 *Tasks: (2.25) sliced meats	4 *Tasks: salads	7 *Tasks: gelatin salads
Average	2 *Tasks: frozen vegetables	5 *Tasks: sandwiches	8 *Tasks: stuffed peppers
High	3 *Tasks: roast meats	6 *Tasks: baked chicken	9 *Tasks: (3) casseroles

Labor Rates (vertical axis label)

*Assign labor factors, reflecting degree of product convenience and level of skilled labor or complexity for similar tasks as shown in each square.

CHAPTER 6
INCREASING PROFITS BY FORECASTING

No matter how well the menu cycle is planned, and despite diligent application of proper pricing strategies, the cafeteria will lose money if the correct quantity of food is not prepared or if it is not prepared in a timely manner so that it is available when customers want to buy it. Overproduction is wasteful and costly, because 100% of the value of leftovers can very seldom be redeemed, no matter how skillfully they are handled. Underproduction can be just as costly if customers are unable to purchase items offered on the menu, because the profit margin of the potential sale is lost and the disappointed customer is one step closer to being lost. To have the fewest leftovers and the fewest unserved customers, the food service administrator must retrieve information on usage from the records and use it to forecast future needs.

The forecasting process, as related to the hospital cafeteria, is the prediction of future sales of food items based on the analysis of the data relating to past sales of food items. In chapter 5, figure 5B, Daily Production Record, and figure 5C, Resale Food Requisition, were introduced as sources of usage information, and the electronic cash register readout was mentioned as a data source. The usage information from these sources concerning daily production items should be retained, ideally as a sales mix analysis as in figure 5A, but at least as a list of items sold on each day of cafeteria operation with a sales mix percent calculation. The nonproduction items, such as those listed on the resale food requisition, figure 5C, do not need to be converted into a sales mix analysis format, as they are stock items that can be used up over the course of several days. For these items, a regular review of the par, or stock, level to ensure that it is adequate is all that is necessary.

For those items that must be accurately forecasted, the sales mix analysis or item list with just the sales mix percent calculation will provide half of the information necessary. The other half needed is customer count information; a record of customer counts should be kept, with the information broken down by sales periods.

Figure 6A is a graphic record of lunch customers during a one-month period. It can readily be seen that the customer count does fluctuate slightly, but the range of fluctuation is tight enough to allow accurate forecasting based on the expectation that the potential customer count can be projected for any given day on the basis of records. It should be noted that figure 6A is a summary of activities for the month of February. The low meal count Monday of one week is the result of Washington's Birthday and the remainder of that week was a school recess period, causing a high number of hospital employees to take vacation at that time and therefore causing lower customer counts than usual throughout the week. The other three weeks' activity should be considered a better base for future forecasting, but the record of activity during a holiday and vacation period is useful during similar periods throughout the year.

Each food item can now be forecasted by multiplying the projected customer count by the sales mix percent for each item. From the information given in figure 6A, it would be reasonable to project a customer count of 315 at lunch on the first Monday following the Mondays charted. If it has been determined, for example, that 21% of all customers will purchase fillet of cod from those items on the menu to be offered on that day, the forecast for fillet of cod would be as follows:

315 projected customers x 21% sales mix = 66 portions forecasted

When this type of forecasting is applied to all menu items to be produced, the food service administrator can be certain that production can profitably be planned for the day's menu.

The forecasting and menu planning process must be done adequately before the day being planned, in order to allow time for production planning. It is not within the scope of this publication to go in depth into the production process, but the information presented is intended to show how the needs of the cafeteria can most accurately be communicated to the production areas so that those needs can be met. The essentials of the production planning process, as it is affected by the cafeteria, are the incorporation of the cafeteria forecasts into the production forecasts generated from other areas, such as the patient area and maybe a coffee shop or vending area.

An ideal production situation exists when the cafeteria's needs require production of additional portions of items scheduled for production but not additional items to be produced. This situation can be achieved by making the cafeteria menu the same as the patient regular diet menu. This approach requires that the menu be well designed and planned and that close attention be paid to usage trends, stock levels, and planning techniques so that the cafeteria will not need to become a run-out area for overproduction food items.

Profit, or whatever the bottom line is expected to show, will be best achieved when the proper amount of food is prepared and sold, without loss, in a well mixed menu that has been priced to yield the expected financial objective. This is not an impossible feat and is not even particularly difficult. However, it does require continuous attention to details such as usage figures and cost/price information, an awareness of what the customer wants to buy and what the food production activity can prepare, and a willingness to make the ongoing adjustments necessary in a planning process of true value.

Figure 6A.
Graph of Cafeteria Lunch Customers, February

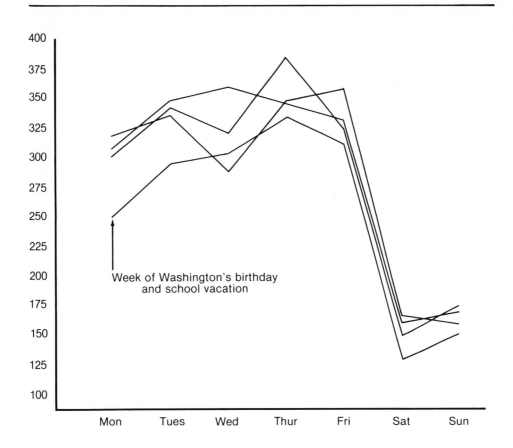

CHAPTER 7
ISSUING FOOD AND SUPPLIES

Any item transferred from one cost center to another needs to be properly accounted for. This requires documentation that provides the name or a description of the item, the unit of issue, and the quantity transferred. Signatures or initials indicating issue and receipt as well as day and date of transfer should be included on the form. Provisions must be made for costing each item, which may be done by using unit price and cost extension columns on the requisition or by a weekly or monthly reconciliation based on a format established by the food service administrator. Issue and acceptance of food or nonfood items from the food service storeroom, cold storage areas, production areas, or the central storeroom of the hospital to the cafeteria should be handled in much the same way that receipts from outside vendors are handled.

The Daily Production Record (figure 5B) was introduced in chapter 5 as a source of usage information and was mentioned in chapter 6 as a forecasting and communications tool. It is also a form of requisition, in that it records those food items requested by the cafeteria and issued by the production areas. If price information from the appropriate standard cost recipes is added, the Daily Production Record becomes a costed requisition. This cost information could be incorporated into the form with the addition of unit price and extension columns, or it could be recorded separately, using the Daily Production Record as an unpriced delivery record and applying the price information to it after it has fulfilled its purpose in the cafeteria and production areas.

The Resale Food Requisition (figure 5C) is an example of a requisition with pricing information on the form itself. After it has been filled out, the requisition is sent to a bookkeeper and the current prices of those items transferred are written in the "Unit Price" column and extended in the "Cost" column. A variation on pricing technique is used with figure 7A, a food requisition, and figure 7B, a nonfood requisition. These forms are computer generated and include a check digit and catalog number in the first column on the left, so that the issuance of each item is identifiable within the program. A reduction of inventory and costing for each item issued is recorded by the computer. This transaction is based on information entered into the computer at the time of receipt from an outside vendor. This process also generates, at certain times established by the hospital food service administrator, a summary of costed requisitions.

Requisitions are necessary for each category of item the cafeteria needs in order to operate. These categories include food, cleaning supplies, service ware, disposables, stationery, and other categories depending on the requirements of each individual cafeteria. Separate and dissimilar requisitions can be used for different categories or subcategories or for different sources of supply, or a standard requisition form can be used for all categories of items and sources of supply, depending on the wishes of the food service administrator. The issuing and requisition system will vary from one hospital to the next. In all cases, however, the cost information on food and supplies must be recorded and identified as a charge to a cost center for proper accountability, review, and analysis.

Figure 7A
Computer-Generated Food Requisition

```
PROGRAM IIS235      S T A N D A R D   R E Q U I S I T I O N            PAGE:     1
DATE ISSUED:                                            ISSUED BY:
DEPARTMENT NO: 006120   DEPARTMENT NAME: FOOD SERVICE                    82/01/12
CATALOG    DESCRIPTION                      ISSUE   REQUESTED        DELIVERED
--------   ----------------------------     ----    ------------     -------------

00 00015   BAKING POWDER                    CAN     ............     ............

00 00017   BAKING SODA                      BOX     ............     ............

00 00020   BEVERAGE CHOCOLATE SYRUP         CASE    ............     ............

00 00024   BEVERAGE COFFEE INSTANT          BOX     ............     ............

00 00025   BEVERAGE COFFEE INSTANT-DECAFE   CASE    ............     ............

00 00028   BEVERAGE FRUIT PUNCH MIX         PKG     ............     ............

00 00030   BEVERAGE 7-UP                    CASE    ............     ............

00 00031   BEVERAGE 7-UP DIETETIC           CASE    ............     ............

00 00034   BEVERAGE GRAPE MIX               PKG     ............     ............

00 00036   BEVERAGE HOT CHOCOLATE           CASE    ............     ............

00 00039   BEVERAGE OVALTINE                JAR     ............     ............

00 00041   BEVERAGE PEPSI                   CASE    ............     ............

00 00042   BEVERAGE PEPSI DIETETIC          CASE    ............     ............

00 00045   BEVERAGE TEA BAGS HOT            CASE    ............     ............

00 00046   BEVERAGE TEA BAGS ICE            CASE    ............     ............

00 00047   BEVERAGE TEA INSTANT ICE         CASE    ............     ............

00 00055   CEREAL BRAN FLAKES               CASE    ............     ............

00 00056   CEREAL, CHEERIOS                 CASE    ............     ............

00 00057   CEREAL CORN FLAKES               CASE    ............     ............

00 00060   CEREAL FARINA                    CASE    ............     ............

00 00063   CEREAL MINI-WHEATS               CASE    ............     ............

00 00065   CEREAL OATMEAL                   BOX     ............     ............

00 00067   CEREAL PUFFED RICE               CASE    ............     ............

00 00069   CEREAL PUFFED WHEAT              CASE    ............     ............

00 00071   CEREAL, RAISIN BRAN              CASE    ............     ............

00 00073   CEREAL RICE KRISPIES             CASE    ............     ............

00 00076   CEREAL SPECIAL K                 CASE    ............     ............

00 00079   CHIFFON BASE & WHIP CHOCOLATE    CASE    ............     ............

00 00080   CHIFFON BASE & WHIP STRAWBERRY   CASE    ............     ............

00 00082   CONDIMENT CATSUP                 CAN     ............     ............

00 00083   CONDIMENT CATSUP P.C.            CASE    ............     ............

00 00086   CONDIMENT CHEESE GRATED          BTL     ............     ............

00 00090   CONDIMENT LEMON JUICE            BTL     ............     ............

00 00094   CONDIMENT MUSTARD                GAL     ............     ............

00 00095   CONDIMENT MUSTARD P.C.           CASE    ............     ............

00 00098   CONDIMENT PAPRIKA                CAN     ............     ............

00 00101   CONDIMENT PEPPER BLACK           CAN     ............     ............

00 00102   CONDIMENT PEPPER PACKETS         CASE    ............     ............
```

Figure 7B.
Computer-Generated Nonfood Requisition

```
PROGRAM IIS235      S T A N D A R D   R E Q U I S I T I O N        PAGE:    8
DATE ISSUED:                                               ISSUED BY:
DEPARTMENT NO: 006120   DEPARTMENT NAME: FOOD SERVICE                81/08/07
CATALOG      DESCRIPTION                     ISSUE   REQUESTED      DELIVERED
--------     ------------------------------  ----   -------------  -------------

02 00136     ISOLATION PLATE BREAD & BUTTER  PKG    .............  .............

02 00139     ISOLATION PLATE DINNER          PKG    .............  .............

02 00140     LID DINNER PLATE                PKG    .............  .............

02 00145     ISOLATION SERVING TRAY          PKG    .............  .............

02 00180     PAPER CHIPS BUTTER              BOX    .............  .............

02 00183     PAPER COASTER 3 1/2 INCH        BOX    .............  .............

02 00196     PAPER CUP BAKING                CASE   .............  .............

02 00210     PAPER CUP 12 OUNCE              TUBE   .............  .............

02 00211     LID PAPER CUP 12 OUNCE          TUBE   .............  .............

02 00220     PAPER DOILIES 6 INCH            BOX    .............  .............

02 00222     PAPER DOILIES 9 INCH            BOX    .............  .............

02 00226     PAPER FREEZER WRAP              ROLL   .............  .............

02 00230     PAPER HAMBURGER PATTY           BOX    .............  .............

02 00235     PAPER PLATE 6 INCH              DOZ    .............  .............

02 00237     PAPER PLATE 9 INCH              DOZ    .............  .............

02 00240     PAPER WAX 9" X 12"              BOX    .............  .............

02 00250     PLASTIC APRON                   BOX    .............  .............

02 00254     PLASTIC BAG SNAP OFF 18X24      CASE   .............  .............

02 00258     PLASTIC BOWL GOLD 8 OUNCE       CASE   .............  .............

02 00259     LID GOLD BOWL                   CASE   .............  .............

02 00263     PLASTIC MUG BROWN 8 OUNCE       CASE   .............  .............

02 00265     PLASTIC MUG GOLD 8 OUNCE        CASE   .............  .............

02 00266     LID MUGS 8 OUNCE                CASE   .............  .............

02 00270     PLASTIC CUP 1 OUNCE             CASE   .............  .............

02 00271     LID CUP 1 OUNCE                 CASE   .............  .............

02 00275     PLASTIC CUP ICE CREAM           CASE   .............  .............

02 00276     LID CUP ICE CREAM               CASE   .............  .............

02 00280     PLASTIC KNIFE                   CASE   .............  .............

02 00281     PLASTIC FORK                    CASE   .............  .............

02 00282     PLASTIC SPOON                   CASE   .............  .............

02 00287     PLASTIC TUMBLER 5 OUNCE         CASE   .............  .............

02 00295     PRINTED NAPKINS                 CASE   .............  .............

02 00297     PRINTED TRAY COVERS             CASE   .............  .............

02 00305     VINYL FILM 6X5                  CASE   .............  .............

02 00306     VINYL FILM 9X9                  CASE   .............  .............

02 00307     VINYL FILM 10X10                CASE   .............  .............

02 00308     VINYL FILM 14X14                CASE   .............  .............

02 00312     VINYL FILM 18X24                ROLL   .............  .............
```

CHAPTER 8
SCHEDULING LABOR

The literature available on the productivity of food service workers indicates that they are about 50% productive, compared with up to 80% productivity in other industries. As the work week shortens and the minimum wage, benefits, and government-mandated costs of employment increase, the cost of a productive hour of labor in the cafeteria will demand more and more sales dollars. The best defense against this inevitably increasing expense is effective, efficient scheduling of employees. To illustrate the importance of this concept, a sample calculation of the cost per productive hour of the lowest-paid cafeteria employee in February 1980 follows:

Base pay	$4.80
FICA (employer's share)	.29
Workers compensation	.10
Unemployment compensation	.14
Medical, hospital, and life insurance	.18
Paid break time (30 minutes)	.32
Vacation (12 days)	.25
Sicktime (10 days)	.21
Holidays (10 days)	.21
Shift differential (2 percent average)	.10
Total cost/paid hour	$6.60

If one multiplies this total by two, assuming that the 50% productivity rate for food service employees is accurate, a productive hour of labor at the base rate costs $13.20. Scheduling labor becomes a most interesting subject after that realization.

THREE APPROACHES

One problem in planning the cafeteria labor schedule is that hospital cafeterias are often scheduled to be open during many hours when there is not enough business to justify the labor needed to operate them. Three basic approaches should be used to resolve this problem to the fullest extent possible:

1. Review the hours of service regularly and become familiar with the cost of staffing a cafeteria during the "valleys" as well as during the "peaks." Then make every effort to eliminate the valleys by closing the cafeteria during those hours. Offering no service except lunch, Monday through Friday, would allow for a highly efficient operation. Although such a

schedule would not allow any hospital cafeteria to serve the hospital staff adequately—the very reason most hospital cafeterias exist—it should be understood that any extension beyond the highest peaks of business jeopardizes productivity. It is possible that a nonessential half-hour or hour could be cut from the hours of service, eliminating some labor. With self-operated vending, as discussed in chapter 12, it is possible that even more unproductive hours could be cut from the schedule, further reducing the need for labor. Although the vast majority of hospitals would be reluctant to make any dramatic change in this scheduling area, some operations may very well benefit from such an approach to containing cafeteria labor cost, either now or in the future.

2. Every effort should be made to smooth out the variance between the peaks and valleys by increasing business during the valleys. The marketing and merchandising ideas presented in chapters 12 and 13 and in part B are a good starting point. If employee meal breaks are rigidly scheduled, there is also the possibility that the peaks could be flattened. If, for instance, all lunch breaks occur from 11:45 a.m. to 1:15 p.m., it may be possible to have that period extended from 11:15 a.m. to 1:45 p.m. This change could be most beneficial in scheduling labor if spreading the number of customers over a longer lunch period would reduce the number of employees required at the peak because of a lower intensity of customers. In this way, the portion of the schedule consumed by the flattened peaks would be a greater percentage of the hours of service. Because people are conditioned to eat at certain times of the day, there are very close limits within which this procedure would work, but it is worth consideration in certain situations.

3. Either of the two preceding approaches will be of some value in making the labor schedule more efficient. However, the major thrust of this chapter is toward the third approach, utilization of an effective system for scheduling labor, discussed by Galya (ref. 5) and Blanken (ref. 6). Effective labor scheduling provides tremendous cost containment potential and is a necessary element of a properly managed cafeteria.

LISTING THE JOBS

The first step in developing a labor schedule is to list the jobs, tasks, or activities that must be performed. Figure 8A is a typical job list, made up of the individual jobs that must be done to operate a cafeteria in accordance with the standards established by the food service administrator. After listing all of the jobs or tasks to be done, the administrator should use work simplification techniques to reduce the amount of time or number of people needed to do the job or to eliminate the job entirely. Some form of time-motion study that the food service administrator can adequately and comfortably work with should be used to provide the data to evaluate each job on the job list.

For example, if dishwashing 6:00 a.m. to 2:30 p.m. was listed as a job and it was determined that from 6:00 a.m. to 8:30 a.m. only a very limited number of dishes were available to be washed, a piece of equipment such as a rack, cart, or pass-through window might allow stacking of dishes so that dishwashing would not have to begin until 7:00 a.m. or later. This would reduce an 8-hour job to a 7-hour job or less. Another possible decision could be that reusable serviceware should be used only at lunch and dinner or not at all. Such a decision would serve to reduce the dishwashing job to a 3-hour part-time job or eliminate it entirely. After every job has been evaluated and refined, improved, or eliminated as necessary, a new job list should be made up of those tasks that will actually be scheduled.

EVALUATING THE JOBS

The jobs that have been determined to be necessary must be evaluated for work content and time consumption. The data collected in the time-motion study can again be used to assign a measurement of work to each job on the list, in order to allow the correct amount of time for completion of each job on the schedule. Also, some jobs—and this may be particularly true in small or not very busy cafeterias—do not require the full attention of an employee. Therefore, although they are valid jobs and may not be changed at all by simplification techniques, they can be done by one employee in tandem with another job or jobs. As an example, operating a grill, making sandwiches, and serving from a steamtable may require at least three employees and even more employees in large cafeterias, but these jobs may all be performed by one employee in certain small cafeterias or at certain times of the day in some cafeterias.

PREPARING THE WORK SCHEDULE

Once simplified and measured jobs have been determined, the actual work schedule can be prepared. The work schedule may be called something else, such as a time-task allocation chart, but essentially it is a chart in bar-graph form that allocates space to every job on the job list. It allows an appropriate amount of time for completion of each job as determined through work measurement and places each job in a proper relationship with every other job and with the cafeteria's scheduled hours of operation.

Figure 8B illustrates a completed cafeteria work schedule. The vertical axis on the left indicates numbered positions, and the horizontal axis represents hours available to be scheduled. After a numbered position has been filled with jobs, ensuring that each job can be completed according to the standard for that job and that an employee assigned to that position will be utilized at optimum efficiency, that position can be assigned to an employee qualified to perform the job in that position. At that point the position becomes a daily activity schedule, a work description, or whatever title might be assigned to a timed listing of the jobs an employee must perform during a shift.

Much trial and error is involved in filling out a work schedule. Figure 8B is completed, but without the jobs filled in or without the positions restricted by beginning and ending times, it is then just a series of horizontal bars, measured by hours, into which all of the jobs on the job list must be fitted. The scheduler's goal is to develop the most compact configuration possible that allocates adequate time for proper performance of each job but does not extend a position beyond the time actually required for that performance. The chart illustrated has nine positions and spans 15 hours, so it could accommodate the scheduling of 135 work hours (9 times 15). As jobs were placed on the schedule, quite a few work hours were assigned. Then, because of work measurement data, the work hours were consolidated.

For example, position 1 is able to perform jobs C, D, E, and WW from 6:00 a.m. to 6:30 p.m., and position 2 is able to perform jobs F, I, J, K, and II from 7:00 a.m. to 9:45 a.m. At the time the cafeteria work schedule in figure 8B was completed, it was determined that the 48 jobs listed in figure 8A could be properly performed with four full-time positions, 1, 2, 4, and 6, and five part-time positions, 3, 5, 7, 8, and 9, amounting to a total of 46.5 work hours (determined by adding the number of hours of work assigned to each position in the cafeteria).

The concept of centralized scheduling, as discussed in chapter 9, is also illustrated in figure 8B. The central scheduler determined that position 3 was needed in the cafeteria only from 10:30 a.m. to 2:00 p.m., but chose not to show it as a part-time position, because a part-time position was available on the kitchen work schedule (not illustrated) from 7:00 a.m. to 10:30 a.m., and there was an hour of work unassigned in the afternoon that could be done from 2:00 p.m. to 3:00 p.m., making a full-time shift. The same idea was applied to position 5, in which the need for two people to work very short shifts in two different areas was combined into a longer part-time shift that could be filled by one employee. Labor cost is charged to each area for the work performed in that area. Position 7 from 12:00 p.m. to 2:30 p.m. and position 8 from 12:00 p.m. to 2:00 p.m. indicate that an employee on another payroll (kitchen) will be assigned to the cafeteria to perform jobs W and V.

CALCULATING THE HOURS AND FTEs PER WEEK

With the transfer of labor for positions 7 and 8 when filled by employees from another area, the cafeteria requires 51 work hours per day on the workday illustrated in figure 8B, 46.5 plus 2.5 (position 7) plus 2 (position 8). On weekends and holidays certain positions may be eliminated from the work schedule to compensate for the lower volume of business. The hours per week and the full-time and part-time positions can be calculated for weekdays as follows:

4 full-time:	30.0 hours/day
5 part-time:	16.5 hours/day
2 assigned part-time:	4.5 hours/day
	51.0 hours/day

51.0 hours/day x 5 days (Mon.-Fri.) = 255 weekday hours/week

On weekends and holidays positions 3 and 4 and the assigned portions of 7 and 8 can be eliminated. The weekend hours are calculated as follows:

Full-time, positions 1, 2, 6:	22.5 hours/weekend day
Part-time, positions 5, 7 (4-7:30 only), 8 (4-7:30 only), 9:	12.0 hours/weekend day
	34.55 hours/weekend day

34.5 hours/day x 2 days (Sat.-Sun.) = 69 hours/weekend

Total weekly work hours are 255 weekday hours plus 69 weekend hours, or 324 required work hours per week.

Positions can be calculated as follows:

4 full-time/weekday x 5 =	20
3 full-time/weekend-day x 2 =	6
	26 full-time shifts/week
5 part-time/weekday x 5 =	25
4 part-time/weekend-day x 2 =	8
2 assigned part-time/weekday x 5	10
	43 part-time shifts/week

For a 37.5-hour workweek the full-time equivalent (FTE) employees required are 324 hours ÷ 37.5 = 8.64 FTE

Although this example is for a cafeteria where employees work 37.5 hours a week, the principles presented apply equally to operations with a shorter or longer workweek. Also, although the example is based on a 5-day workweek, a 4-day workweek could be planned in exactly the same manner.

PREPARING THE EMPLOYEE SCHEDULE

The information developed to this point is the raw data necessary before the scheduler can make out an employee schedule that will list employees by name and the shifts they are to work. The number of employees to be used to cover the example work schedule could vary depending on the workweek, the pay period, and the weekend policies of each individual hospital, as well as the full-time and part-time employees available. The cafeteria work schedule illustrated could be covered with all part-time employees, some of them working full-time shifts four or fewer days per week, but in no case with more than five full-time employees (26 shifts divided by 5 days per workweek), with at least one part-time employee to work the remaining full-time shift.

The development of an optimum schedule for cafeteria labor should be a totally objective process. Individual employees, with their individual strengths, weaknesses, likes, and dislikes, become a part of the schedule only after the preceding steps have been taken to determine the real needs of the cafeteria and the demand that those needs will place on employees when they are assigned to the positions in the cafeteria.

Figure 8A.
Job List

A. Pick up breakfast food and pastry from kitchen

B. Set food up on serving line

C. Make coffee

D. Set up other beverages

E. Set up cash register

F. Serve hot breakfast 6:30 a.m.- 11 a.m.

G. Take cash 6:30 a.m.-11:00 a.m.

H. Wash dishes 6:30 a.m.-7:00 p.m.

I. Set up condiment counter

J. Set up salad bar

K. Set up sandwich bars (2)

L. Set up salad counter

M. Set up dessert counter

N. Operate grill 11:30 a.m.-1:30 p.m.

O. Serve from steamtable 11:30 a.m.- 1:30 p.m.

P. Stock salad counter 11:30 a.m.- 1:30 p.m.

Q. Stock dessert counter 11:30 a.m.- 1:30 p.m.

R. Take cash 11:30 a.m.-2:00 p.m.

S. Take cash 2:00 p.m.-4:00 p.m.

T. Take cash 5:00 p.m.-7:00 p.m.

U. Second dishwasher 12:00 p.m.- 2:30 p.m.

V. Food runner 11:00 a.m.-1:30 p.m.

W. Third dishwasher 12:30 p.m.- 1:30 p.m.

Y. Mop floors and take out garbage a.m.

Z. Mop floors and take out garbage early p.m.

AA. Mop floors and take out garbage late p.m.

BB. Clean dining room tables a.m.

CC. Clean dining room tables p.m.

DD. Food runner 4:30 p.m.-7:00 p.m.

EE. Serve from steam table 5:00 p.m.-7:00 p.m.

FF. Operate grill 4:30 p.m.-7:00 p.m.

GG. Stock salad counter 4:30 p.m.- 7:00 p.m.

HH. Stock dessert counter 4:30 p.m.- 7:00 p.m.

II. Clean up grill a.m.

JJ. Clean up grill early p.m.

KK. Clean up grill late p.m.

LL. Clean up salad/sandwich bar after 1:30 p.m.

MM. Set up popcorn machine before 2:00 p.m.

NN. Clean up popcorn machine after 4:00 p.m.

OO. Clean dishmachine a.m.

PP. Clean dishmachine early p.m.

QQ. Clean dishmachine late p.m.

RR. Clean steamtable/serving area late p.m.

SS. Inventory and order food and supplies

TT. Prepare cash deposit 11:00 a.m.

UU. Prepare cash deposit 2:00 p.m.

VV. Prepare cash deposit 7:00 p.m.

WW. Supervise employees 6:00 a.m.- 7:30 p.m.

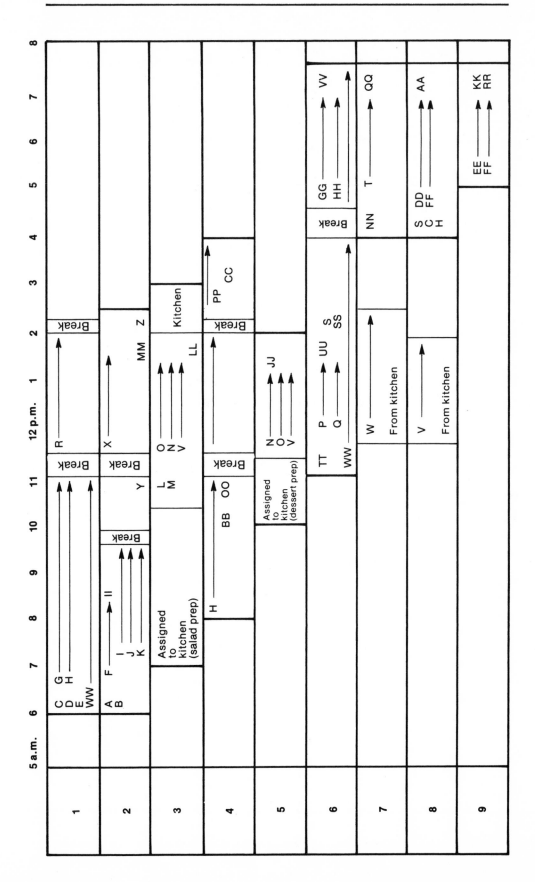

CHAPTER 9
FACTORS AFFECTING PRODUCTIVITY

It is probably safe to say that no two hospital cafeterias in the world are exactly alike. Further, school and college cafeterias, business and industry cafeterias, nursing home cafeterias, military cafeterias, and public cafeterias all differ to varying degrees. It only stands to reason, therefore, that somewhere someone is running a better cafeteria. There are cafeterias with better systems, better designs, better menus, better service, and happier customers. All of those better things mean that there are opportunities for all food service administrators to make improvements in the cafeterias they manage, and being accountable for the cafeteria operation assigns the responsibility to administrators to seek improvement actively and constantly. Such a search requires administrators to read books and trade journals, to join professional associations such as the American Society for Hospital Food Service Administrators (ASHFSA), to make site visits to other operations, and to maintain an objective view of the possibilities available. Some of the major and most obvious considerations for further exploration are the following:

CENTRALIZATION

Centralization of systems should be researched, and methods to implement centralization should be developed. In general, the more a function can be centralized, the more productive it will become. The functions listed below can each be divided into three steps—preparation, performance, and cleanup. The preparation and cleanup steps are unproductive, and the only productive step is performance. Therefore the most performance that can be obtained without adding more preparation and cleanup yields the greatest productivity. More time devoted to the productive performance of a function relative to the necessary unproductive steps is the impetus for centralization. More efficient utilization of equipment and tighter supervision made possible by the less sprawling nature of the function may also result from centralization. The following functions should be considered:

- *Menu.* The cafeteria menu and the patient menu can be exactly the same, except for modified diets, offering patients a menu good enough to attract cafeteria customers, who are not a captive audience, and offering cafeteria customers a menu good enough for patients, the most important people in the hospital. This step may require some modification of the existing menus, but it will pay off by eliminating all the time, both productive and unproductive, required to offer the additional items available on two uncoordinated menus.

- *Production.* Centralized production is most beneficial if the menus have also been centralized. Even without menu centralization, the production function should be centralized to limit the purchase of expensive equipment and to minimize the number of highly trained and more expensive production employees necessary in the operation. Also, decentralized production requires space, additional raw product storage and availability, either more supervisors or less intense supervision, and duplicated preparation and cleanup.

- *Ingredients.* A major subsystem of the production function is the preparation of ingredients. In recent years the concept of separate preparation and measuring of ingredients in an "ingredient room" apart from the production area has been developed. Although the concept is based in part on using less expensive labor in the ingredient room to perform preparation steps, rather than more expensive cooks who are paid according to their ability to perform production steps, the ingredient room is primarily a centralization of a subsystem. Imagine a day's menu with four recipes calling for chopped celery. Without the ingredient room, four trips would be made to the refrigerator to get the celery, four cleaning, cutting, and measuring processes would go on, four equipment cleaning processes would go on, and four trips back to the refrigerator to return the amount not used would be made—all by a highly paid cook. With a centralized ingredient room, a lower-paid employee would prepare all the chopped celery needed for all the recipes being used that day or for several days. The only steps that would take place more than once would be measuring. This procedure would obviously increase the rate of productivity.

- *Warewashing.* Space and equipment costs alone make centralized warewashing more attractive than decentralized warewashing. No warewashing machine works without at least one employee operating it, and most machines used in hospitals require two to six or more employees to operate at peak capacity. Accordingly, any operation that has more than one warewashing area, machine, and staff has the potential to increase productivity by centralizing that function. In some hospitals, however, the cafeteria and patient warewashing areas are so far apart that centralized warewashing is not feasible. Therefore, an in-depth cost analysis should be done prior to a change in the warewashing function.

- *Scheduling of personnel.* Shift overlaps in one area do not necessarily correspond to shift overlaps or peak demands in another area. Therefore, flexibility in scheduling employees in several different areas is most attractive. This flexibility can be best accomplished when the scheduling process is centralized, so that the needs of the entire department and the employees available to fill those needs can be evaluated by one scheduler. Labor scheduling is discussed in detail in chapter 8.

- *Food service systems.* The benefits of centralizing food service functions and improving the efficiency, quality, and effectiveness of a food service system have been demonstrated by Kaud (ref. 7). These changes contributed significantly to improvement in productivity and to the reduction of total food service department costs. Ball and Durfee (ref. 8) have shown that a change in a food service delivery system increased productivity, decreased cost, and improved the quality of patient care. Crum (ref. 9) delineated the effects of a health care facility merger on productivity improvement and innovation in a food service department.

VENDING MACHINES

The purchase or leasing and operation of vending machines should be considered. Self-operated vending by the food service department can be a highly productive and profitable extension of the manual food service that exists. Vending is discussed in detail in chapter 12.

SERVICEWARE

The decision to use disposable serviceware or reusable serviceware affects productivity. A reevaluation of the cafeteria's position should be made each time the warewashing machine needs replacement and each time food service employees receive a pay increase. Aesthetic questions aside, the determining factors are the condition and cost of equipment, the availability of storage and sanitizing space, the cost of refuse removal, and the cost of labor. With expensive labor, disposables can lower costs if the number of employees can, in fact, be lowered. If for some reason the number of employees would not change with either system, reusable serviceware could well be less expensive. There is no universal answer to the disposable or reusable serviceware question, and an in-depth cost analysis must be made to evaluate the alternatives accurately and to reevaluate them as suggested above.

MAINTENANCE AND REPAIR

An unfortunate trend in the food service business seems to be the lack of good on-site maintenance and repair of equipment and little or no preventive maintenance. Operating a cafeteria, or any food operation, requires adequate working equipment kept in good repair. A hamburger cannot be sold if the grill lacks a heating element, and the profit on a soft drink will not be realized if the carbonator is broken. It is up to the food service administrator to develop and follow through on a preventive maintenance program for all equipment and to review the equipment with the people who use it to make sure that it is properly used and that it remains adequate for the job.

Because of the increasingly sophisticated nature of food service equipment, a list of outside, factory-authorized service agencies and the equipment they will service should be maintained. Service contracts with these agencies should be explored, and in some cases preventive maintenance contracts can be established. Furthermore, some food service purveyors such as coffee and postmix soft drink companies offer their product at a price that includes regular preventive maintenance on equipment. In most situations, this type of arrangement has worked well and to the benefit of the hospital.

EQUIPMENT PURCHASE

The food service administrator must purchase, or at least request the purchase of, new and more sophisticated equipment as it becomes available and is needed. Any equipment purchase will, of course, cost money, but if the money isn't spent for needed equipment the department will not have the tools necessary to operate the cafeteria properly and, in time, the lost productivity and/or sales will cost more than the purchase of the equipment needed. Rejections of proposals to purchase equipment would be reduced if the food service administrator would objectively justify the purchase prior to presenting the proposal to higher authority.

Again, an in-depth cost/benefit analysis is necessary. Why is the existing piece of equipment, if such exists, no longer adequate? Is it fully depreciated? How much will the new equipment cost installed and will there be any expense incurred in removing the old equipment? What is the projected life of the new equipment? Who will service it? Why is it needed? Does it perform a necessary function, simplify the performance of function, or will it be used to perform a new function? Why is that function necessary and what will be the benefit of performing it? If the equipment is a replacement, is the function it performs still necessary, and why? What alternatives have been considered? Only after satisfactorily answering these questions should the food service administrator present the proposal for equipment purchase to hospital administration, reinforced by the factual information developed in those answers.

A productive cafeteria is easier to operate than an underproductive one, because many of the problems encountered by food service administrators can be related to the factors affecting productivity discussed above. By taking the necessary steps to ensure productive menu planning, food production, ingredient preparation, warewashing, and employee scheduling and by providing the right services, using the most suitable serviceware, and having adequate equipment in good repair, much of the crisis management is taken out of the operation of the cafeteria, and more time can be devoted to the more productive management by objectives.

CHAPTER 10
CASH CONTROLS
AND SECURITY PROCEDURES

One of the pleasures of a cafeteria operation is the immediate cash payment for the sale of food and service. Cash sales provide an immediate feedback on the effect of a change in menu, service, or price and can give immediate satisfaction when an increase in cash sales results from a special promotion in the cafeteria. Although cash sales offer immediate feedback on your cafeteria service, perhaps positive or negative, cash also demands security, control, and analysis of when, where, how, and for what it has been collected.

The food service administrator cannot personally handle the cash sales in the cafeteria, as that is a full-time job. Nevertheless, ultimate responsibility for sales and cash comes back to that office. The food service administrator must, therefore, do all the following:

- Keep all money locked in a secure safe when it is not actively being received into a cash register or being used as part of a cashier's working bank. The combination should be known only by those who absolutely need to know it. In a large, busy cafeteria pickups may be made by a supervisor and signed for and deposited in the safe each time a cashier accumulates $200 (or any other amount felt to be appropriate) in 10-dollar and 20-dollar bills. The less money held in the least secure position (the cash register) and the more money held in the most secure position (the bank), with the safe falling somewhere in between but closer to the cash register, the more secure the money will be.

- Deposit receipts daily (Monday through Friday). Do not deposit them at exactly the same time every day or take exactly the same route to the bank each trip. (The bank may be any point at which a valid receipt is received for the money and the responsibility for its security is transferred from the food service department).

- Control the safe with a log that must be signed, dated, and timed at each entry. Each withdrawal must be signed for, whether it is a bank deposit to be made by a member of management or the checkout of a working bank by a cashier. The date, time, and amount should be noted, and the amount withdrawn or deposited should be verified.

- Throw away the clear keys for the cash register. The primary means of checking a cashier is by comparing cash receipts with cash register readings. Clearing the cumulative reading will nullify the comparison and is never really necessary.

- Allow only one cashier to operate a register between reconciliations. Hold each cashier responsible for the reconciliation, but don't expect anyone to accept responsiility if more than one person has been allowed to enter the same cash drawer without a full accounting at each change of cashiers.
- Avoid allowing a cashier to see the beginning and ending readings prior to depositing the money. All money in the cash drawer should be turned in, with receipt acknowledged. Then, in the presence of the cashier, the amount that was turned in, less the bank, should be compared to the difference between the beginning and ending readings.
- Conduct surprise audits. Walk up to a cash register, ask the cashier to remove all money, read the register, then conduct the normal reconciliation procedure. Do this when least expected, such as at the peak of the lunchtime rush. Merely supply a substitute cashier and cash drawer for the course of the audit, then take register readings upon returning the cashier who was audited to the register.

VERIFYING CASH SALES

Cash sales can most easily and regularly be verified through the use of a form such as the cafeteria cash report (see figure 10A). The cash report illustrated shows management interest in sales for the five distinct periods of the day. The report also shows total sales for the day, customer counts, deposits, cash breakdown at the time of deposit, and the cashier and supervisor responsible for each period of sales.

The beginning "X key" reading and customer count reading are entered on line B just prior to opening at 6:30 a.m. At 9:00 a.m., the breakfast sales period is ended, and coffee breaks or snack sales begin. The 9:00 a.m. "X key" reading and customer count reading are posted on line A, the ending reading for breakfast, and on line E, the beginning reading for snack sales. Subtracting line B from line A shows the sales recorded and the number of customer transactions recorded during the period between the two readings. The cashier on duty and the supervisor who took the readings initial the "Audit" column, indicating responsibility for the figures reported. At 11:00 a.m. the "X key" reading and customer count reading are posted on line D, the ending reading for snack sales, and on line I, the beginning reading for lunch sales. Subtracting line E from line D shows the sales recorded and the number of customer transactions recorded during the period between the two readings. Adding line C and line F yields line G, which is the total sales and customer count from 6:00 a.m. to 11:00 a.m., the period for which the first deposit is made.

At 11:00 a.m. a deposit is made up for morning sales. All cash is taken from the register and counted, using lines U through Z, which form a cash count sheet. The total from line Z is entered on line D in the "Deposit" column; the amount of the cashier's bank is entered on line E and subtracted from line D to yield line F, the deposit. Line F in the "Deposit" column is compared to line G in the "Cash" column to arrive at the amount over or short for the period. Appropriate initials in the "Audit" column indicate responsibility. The "Reset" box is used only if the cash register is cleared, a procedure not recommended. The remainder of the day's sales are recorded in the same basic manner, taking readings and entering them where indicated, and counting money for deposit where indicated. The entire day is summarized by adding lines G, K, and R in the "Count" and "Cash" columns and by adding lines F, J, and Q in the "Deposit" column. This summary is entered on line S.

The form illustrated in figure 10A is for one specific operation. The times that readings are taken, the sales categories, and the times that deposits are made will differ from cafeteria to cafeteria. Obviously, a deposit must be made each time a cashier goes off duty. With minor changes to fit any cafeteria's needs, this cash report will give complete information, with a basis for continuity (ref. 10). Figure 10A was designed to record cash sales only, not other sales categories, thereby making it possible to condense the number of cash reports required into one report per cash register per day. There are many acceptable formats for cash register reconciliation and sales data accumulation. It is most important, however, that the basic principles of cash control be incorporated into whatever format is chosen or designed by the hospital food service administrator.

The cash reports should be accumulated and summarized weekly or monthly. A weekly summary could be an extension of the format for the daily report. A monthly summarization (see figure 10B) is merely a form for the transfer and summarization of the information generated by the daily reports (ref. 11).

COMPARING SALES AND CONSUMPTION

With a good breakdown of sales at hand, it then becomes interesting to compare those sales to the food consumed, as shown by requisitions and production sheets. For the increasing number of food service administrators who have electronic preset cash registers in the cafeteria, this is a simple process that is explained in the register's operating manual. For those with manual or standard electric registers, this comparison requires a bit more work, but it can nonetheless be done fairly accurately. The most basic level of sales comparison is done by having the cashier record by hand the number of an item or items sold. Then these totals are compared to the number of that item or items the kitchen recorded as having sent to the cafeteria, minus overproduction.

Some electric registers have department or function keys, which can be used to record the sales of specific items on an audit basis. At breakfast one morning all doughnuts might be rung on key A, all Danish pastries on key B, and so forth, through the number of keys available. At the end of breakfast the sales recorded on key A should equal the value of the doughnuts depleted from inventory multiplied by the selling price, key B should equal the value of Danish pastries used, and so forth. At lunchtime, those keys can be used to record sales for different items and at dinner for still different items, or a key could be used to record sales of one specific item for a whole day. This procedure will be most effective if only the food service administrator and the cashiers know which items are being recorded by this means.

The most difficult sales comparison without an electronic register is an audit of all food sold over an extended period such as a week. By accumulating every requisition and extending and totaling them, an exact value of food sent to the cafeteria during the period can be determined. By comparing the total requisitioned value to total sales, the exact food cost for the period can be determined as a percentage of sales. By extending each requisition into sales value, adjusting for inventory variance, and comparing it to recorded sales, a loss factor can be determined, which will either indicate that what the kitchen sends to the cafeteria is properly sold or that there is a need for further investigation.

An electronic cash register with preset keys can provide the above sales information as frequently as needed. Each department key, as it is depressed to record a sale, accumulates sales data. Reading a manual or standard electric register provides only total sales and a few department totals, but reading an electronic register can provide sales data from each of up to 200 or more department (item) keys in essentially the same amount of time, with no more work than reading the standard register. Audits and analyses become routine with electronic registers, rather than the occasional chores they are with manual or standard electric cash registers.

The cash register is more than just a machine for ringing up sales and storing money. Analyzing the information provided by the register presents an opportunity to review the quantity of food forecasted, produced, requisitioned, and sold. A variance between the number of items indicated as sold by the cash register and the number supplied as indicated by production sheets and requisitions could be due to theft, overportioning or underportioning, recipe shrinkage, or inaccurately kept records. In any of these cases, the need for action by management is signaled by the cafeteria's cash control and security procedures.

CATERING

A discussion of cash controls and security procedures is not complete without addressing one of the cafeteria's most controversial topics, the catering function. It is not the purpose of this publication to discuss the varied issues associated with the principle of catering foods to a hospital's board of directors and departments; however, the aim is to provide a mechanism to identify this function clearly for proper accounting purposes. To strengthen the accountability of the cafeteria catering activities and to identify the magnitude and the scope of this service, a cafeteria catering order (see figure 10C) is recommended. The cafeteria catering order identifies the essential information required for: (1) function, date and time of service, location, and number of guests; (2) name of the person or department ordering the catering service, justification for the order and appropriate (designated) administrative approval; (3) menu description and cost; and (4) billing information. Justification or administrative approval is not required when the catering function is paid for in cash or by a personal check. The cafeteria catering order is prepared in triplicate. The first copy is given to the customer, the second copy is forwarded to fiscal affairs, and the third copy is retained in the cafeteria for its records.

To maintain accountability for the cafeteria catering functions, each cafeteria catering order is serially numbered. When a catering is served, the total amount of the catering is rung up on the register either as a cash or charge sale, and the fiscal affairs copy of the cafeteria catering order is included in the register sale. In addition, a record should be kept to provide an audit trail of all the cafeteria catering order requests in a numerical sequence.

Figure 10A.
Cafeteria Cash Report

Day _____ Date _____

	Time	Reading	Count	Cash	Instruction	Deposit	Audit
A	9 a.m.	Ending					Cshr
B	6:30 a.m.	- Beginning					Cshr
C		= Breakfast sales					Spvr
D	11 a.m.	Ending			Cash		Cshr
E	9 a.m.	- Beginning			- Bank		Cshr
F		= A.M. snack sales			= Deposit		Spvr
G		C & F = Subtotal			Over/(short)		Reset
H	2 p.m.	Ending			Cash		Cshr
I	11 a.m.	- Beginning			- Bank		Cshr
J		= Lunch sales			= Deposit		Spvr
K		J = Subtotal			Over/(short)		Reset
L	5 p.m.	Ending					Cshr
M	2 p.m.	- Beginning					Cshr
N		= P.M. snack sales					Spvr
O	6:30 p.m.	Ending			Cash		Cshr
P	5 p.m.	- Beginning			- Bank		Cshr
Q		= Dinner sales			= Deposit		Spvr
R		N & Q = subtotal			Over/(short)		Reset
S		G + K + R = Total sales			F + J + Q =		Total deposit

		11:00 a.m.	2:00 p.m.	6:30 p.m.	
T	$				Comments:
U	Bills				
V	Q				
W	D				
X	N				
Y	P				
Z	Total				

Figure 10B.
Monthly Summary of Cafeteria Sales Report

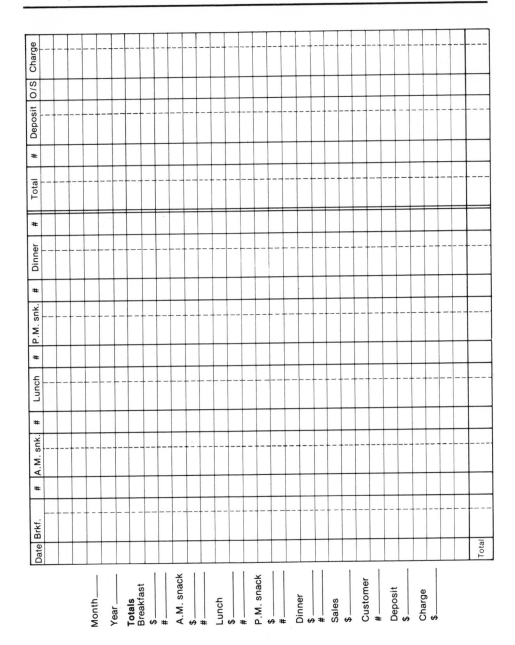

Figure 10C.
Cafeteria Catering Order

CAFETERIA CATERING ORDER
(3-Day Advance Reservation Required)

No.　9765

Function _____

Date of Service _____ Delivery Time _____

Location _____ Guests _____

Requested by _____ Telephone _____ Date _____

Justification: _____

_____

_____

Administrative Approval _____

Quantity	Item	Unit	Total
		Catering Fee	
		Total Amount	

Billing Information　　　　**Coding**

☐ Hospital Department　　　Unit Division Dept.

☐ Other Department　　　Unit-Division-Dept.　Requisition No.

☐ Nonhospital Organization　　　Address

CUSTOMER

FISCAL AFFAIRS

CAFETERIA

Reprinted with permission of University of Wisconsin Hospital and Clinics.

CHAPTER 11
THE OPERATING STATEMENT

A review of the literature indicates a myriad of operating statements in use in the health care field, with the format varying significantly from hospital to hospital.

A typical hospital cafeteria operating statement may have these major components: income; direct expenses broken into food, labor, supply, and other expenses; total direct expenses; indirect expenses; and profit or loss from operation. The operating statement may show the name of the health care institution, cost center, the period of operation, budgeted expenditure, and variances between actual operation and budgeted performance. This information is extended to show year-to-date experience. In addition, operating statements may show productivity indicators and statistical information. Examples of operating statements and supplementary schedules are furnished by Kaud (ref. 12). The supplementary schedules cover information on personnel, food expense, supply expense, and other expenses. These direct expenses are incurred while conducting the planned performance of an activity or a cost center. Those expenses that cannot be clearly assigned to a cost center, such as heat, light, air conditioning, building depreciation, and accounting costs, are classified as indirect costs. If the objective of a health care institution is to break even in the cafeteria, indirect costs need to be included as well as direct costs of food, labor, supply, and other expenses.

Thus, when a cafeteria operating statement features detailed financial information, it serves as an excellent managerial tool for the food service administrator because it captures the essential information necessary for the management of a successful operation.

MEASURING FINANCIAL PERFORMANCE

In an attempt to measure the financial performance of a cafeteria, a well defined procedure has to be in place. Traditionally, a unit of measure is used to determine the soundness of an operation. This measure consists of two major components, output and input.

The output in the cafeteria may be identified as sales (dollars), number of meal equivalents, average check, or number of customers served. *Sales* are dollars rung up on a cash register, collected in a vending machine coin box, received as a lump-sum payment for a catered function, or sums credited to the nonpatient account and charged to another activity. The *number of meal equivalents* is determined by dividing total cafeteria sales (cafeteria, catering, vending machines, and so forth) by the average selling price of a full meal served at noon. (A full meal consists of an entree, vegetable, potato, salad, dessert, and beverage.) This average selling price is the value of the meal equivalent. *Average check* is arrived at by dividing total sales by the cafeteria customer count. The *number of customers served* is obtained by recording the number of transactions from the cash register and counting the number of guests served by catered functions.

The input is defined as the employment of the necessary resources to produce the output. The input may be identified as dollars invested and/or as number of hours either worked or paid. *Number of hours worked* is associated with productive hours, but *hours paid* reflects total hours worked plus benefit hours, usually totaling forty hours per week, for full-time employment. The benefit hours are better known as nonproductive hours, such as vacation, sick leave, and other paid benefit days or hours.

Generally, the dollars expended for fringe benefits may include FICA, medical insurance premiums, unemployment compensation, worker's compensation, and so forth. Further refinements of the number of hours may include a breakdown of management hours and all nonsalaried hours such as production, service, and janitorial services. The total of these hours is calculated to produce the number of full-time equivalent (FTE) employees (40 hours per week times 52 weeks equals 2,080 hours per year) and is differentiated by worked or paid hours or minutes, to be used in the financial evaluation of the cafeteria.

A one-month operating statement for a hospital cafeteria is presented in figure 11A as a case study for analysis. The objective of this cafeteria is to break even after paying from income for food, labor, supplies, other direct costs, and indirect costs. After an analysis of the statement in relation to the cafeteria's goals, recommendations are made to improve the financial operation of the cafeteria.

As a first step in close examination of the financial data, costs are examined in relation to income in order to highlight any area of weakness. The costs are expressed as a percentage of total sales, as shown in figure 11A. Food costs represent 51%, labor costs represent 42%, other expenses represent 6%, and net profit represents 1%. The combined food and labor costs amount to 93% of total income. At a glance, it is apparent that the combined food and labor costs are excessive. These two areas require further analysis to ascertain how to correct this situation.

To continue the analysis of the cafeteria operation, the number of meal equivalents has to be determined. The purpose of determining the number of meal equivalents is to establish the percentage of patient and nonpatient food service activities and to allocate operating costs accordingly. The number of meal equivalents served is affected by the value set for the meal equivalent. As an example, figure 11B, Value of Meal Equivalent Calculation, shows the number of meal equivalents when three different values are assigned: $2.00, $2.25, and $2.50. The average check, based on total income and customer count, is 84 cents. Figure 11B illustrates that the lower the value of the meal equivalent, the higher the number of meal equivalents served.

Figure 11C, Cost per Meal Analysis, shows the impact of the three different values of meal equivalent on the cost of food, labor, other expenses, indirect cost, and profit or loss. Using the same percentages of 51% for food, 42% for labor, and 6% for other expenses, the total direct cost of the meal equivalent will vary depending on the value assigned to the meal equivalent, but the total direct costs will still equal 99% of income. However, when indirect costs of 12% of income are added, a net loss occurs in every calculation. Because the 12% is the recommended level to be budgeted for indirect costs, this calculation confirms that the cost of food and labor is too high. To improve the financial condition of this operation, expenditures for direct costs and indirect costs have to meet the objectives outlined in figure 11C under the column "Break-Even Hospital."

Other items on the operating statement also need adjustment. A close examination of the total labor cost of $21,762 shown in figure 11A discloses that employee fringe benefit expenses are not included in this total. Thus, the cost of labor in this operation is understated by between 15% to 20%. Finally, the scope of the expenses listed under the general heading "Other Expenses" is limited and understated, because those accounts that are traditionally associated with cafeteria operation, such as depreciation, forms and menus, insurance, laundry and uniforms, office supplies, telephone, and repairs, are not covered. Under this same category, "Other Expenses," the amount of soaps and chemicals used is high for a cafeteria service on disposables.

REVIEW OF PRODUCTIVITY

One element of performance standard is the measure of meals per paid hour. Figure 11D, Productivity Indicators, outlines the productivity rate of the cafeteria by the performance standard of number of meal equivalents per paid hour and number of meal equivalents per full-time equivalent (FTE) under three different meal values. A review of the productivity rate appears to be good under the $2.00, fair under the $2.25, and from fair to poor under the $2.50, particularly if the operation utilizes disposables. This evaluation is made on the basis of the assumption that the paid hours are a true representation of paid hours for management, production, service, janitorial, and other related hours.

In addition, the total hours expended in the cafeteria have exceeded the budgeted hours by 4% (see figure 11A). Productive hours of 3,091.2 plus nonproductive hours of 210.4 equal 3,301.6 paid hours, or 19.08 FTE, but budgeted hours of 18.4 FTE times 173 hours per month equal 3,183.2 hours.

Other measures of performance may include the following indicators:

Number of customer transactions/FTE=3,272
Sales/FTE=$2,743
Sales less direct expenses/FTE=$27.31
   ($521 net profit ÷ 19.08 FTE)

The sales information indicates that each FTE contributes 1% to indirect costs, as $27.31 is approximately 1% of $2,743. This confirms the information in figure 11A, that 99% of costs are for direct expenses, with 1% remaining as a contribution to indirect costs.

For the food service administrator to break even in the cafeteria, however, a minimum of 12% of sales is required to meet the indirect costs. This estimate may vary from one institution to another, but the 12% figure is considered adequate to meet the costs associated with indirect expenses for a cafeteria operation.

ANALYSIS OF SALES

Another important aspect of examining the cafeteria operating statement is an in-depth analysis of sales and menu. The information required to accomplish this study is normally not contained in the operating statement but is usually available in the cafeteria records. The food service administrator writes the menu, setting in motion a number of expensive activities, including purchasing, receiving, storage, preparation, cooking, portioning, and service. Since these functions are expensive to perform, the food service administrator predicts that all items carried on the menu are popular with customers and will sell well. To ensure continued success in marketing techniques and an increase in sales, an analysis of sales and labor cost per meal is needed (see figure 11E). This information will be of great value in scheduling employees, determining cafeteria hours, and forecasting meals. Because the cafeteria operation is a complex one, additional detailed sales information is required for efficient use of resources.

The daily sales (menu) record captures the daily menu, food cost, and sales per individual entree item (see figure 11F). The necessary information to complete the number of each entree served and total sales can be easily obtained from electronic cash registers now available on the market. This information is considered essential in cafeteria management for obvious reasons such as planning, forecasting, and scheduling of production and personnel.

RECOMMENDATIONS FOR IMPROVING
THE OPERATING STATEMENT

The food service administrator who is paying attention to consumer trends knows that consumers' style of eating is changing, their taste has become more sophisticated, and they have learned to expect more for their money than ever before. Consumers will not put up with indifferent treatment by service personnel, and they are beginning to know the difference between food that is merely acceptable and food that is superior. Moreover, consumers are very concerned about nutrition and their health. Their selection of food is based on their perception of good, eye-appealing, and nutritious food that will help them maintain their ideal physical fitness. Consumers will continue to be price and value conscious and will be willing to pay for high-quality food. Therefore, the following recommendations are made to improve the cafeteria operation:

1. *Increased sales.* The food service administrator must first concentrate on developing a set of menus that will be perceived by the consumer as nutritious and of high value. This function could be accomplished easily by surveying consumer opinions, needs, and suggestions. This information could serve as a foundation for the change. The daily sales analysis (figure 11E) and the daily sales record (figure 11F) provide the necessary

managerial tools to apply the consumer suggestions and to contribute to meeting indirect cost and the break-even objective.

2. *Food cost.* In spite of rising food prices, cafeteria food cost should be maintained at around 40% of sales or less, depending on the institution's financial objectives. The food service administrator may consider some of these suggestions to improve food cost:
   a. Tighter controls in food preparation and portioning
   b. Efficient purchasing practices
   c. Contract buying to defray some costs
   d. Changes in menu mixes
   e. Menu flexibility
   f. Lower cost menu items
   g. Nonbeef items
   h. New items
   i. Smaller portions
   j. Tighter food control
   k. Minimization of food waste in preparation, cooking, and service
   l. Increase in menu prices
   m. Increase in portion size, addition of other ingredients, and increase in price
   n. Comparison of sales with forecasted food portions
   o. Maintenance of high-quality food at fair value

3. *Labor cost.* To maintain labor cost at 38% of sales, food service administrators are turning to prepared foods, automation, and self-service. Before these alternatives are put into effect, the following subjects need to be explored:
   a. Better labor schedules
   b. Preparation of in-house precooked portion food
   c. Automated, mechanized, and centralized functions
   d. Self-service activities such as a salad bar
   e. Improved productivity

4. *Other expenses.* The role of disposables should be reviewed and their cost accurately ascertained to determine whether disposables are cost-effective. The use of soaps and chemicals should be controlled. Purchasing procedures, including the bidding process for all supply items, should be reviewed.

5. *Indirect cost.* When pricing the menu, the food service administrator should allocate a minimum of 12% to indirect cost, which includes expenses for heat, light, air conditioning, maintenance, and so forth. This practice will account for the full cost of operation and will allow for better understanding of cost and its influence on the menu and on service.

Figure 11A.
Cafeteria Operating Statement, January

Income

Cafeteria		$49,267
Catering		3,070
	Total income	$52,337

Expenses

Food

Meat		8,058	
Dairy		4,103	
Storeroom		8,392	
Fruits/vegetables		2,686	
Other		3,429	
	Total food	$26,668	51%

Labor

Salaries		20,605	
FICA		1,157	
	Total labor	$21,762	42%

Other Expenses

Paper disposables		2,487	5%
Utilities		148	
Soaps/chemicals		112	} 1%
Housekeeping		400	
Miscellaneous		239	
	Total other expenses	$ 3,386	6%
	Net profit (loss)	$ 521	1%

Statistical information:

Cafeteria customer count	$59,358	FTEs	18.4 (budgeted)
Average check	.83	Productive man-hours	3091.2
Catering customer count	3,070	Nonproductive man-hours	210.4

Figure 11B.
Value of Meal Equivalent Calculation

Total income	$52,337	$52,337	$52,337	$52,337
Value of meal equivalent	$2.00	$2.25	$2.50	
Meals/month	26,169	23,261	20,935	
Average meals/day	872	775	698	
Customer count				62,428
Average check				$0.84

Figure 11C.
Cost per Meal Analysis

	Income						Average Check, $ .84		Break-Even Hospital, 100%
	$2.00		$2.25		$2.50				
Food	1.02	51%	1.15	51%	1.27	51%	.43	51%	42%
Labor	.83	42%	.94	42%	1.04	42%	.35	42%	38%
Other expenses	.13	6%	.14	6%	.16	6%	.05	6%	8%
Total direct cost	1.98	99%	2.23	99%	2.47	99%	.83	99%	88%
Indirect cost	.24	12%	.27	12%	.30	12%	.10	12%	12%
Total cost	$2.22	111%	$2.50	111%	$2.77	111%	.93	111%	100%
Net Loss	.22	11%	.25	11%	.27	11%	.09	11%	0

Figure 11D.
Productivity Indicators

Value of meal equivalent	$ 2.00	$2.25	$2.50
Meal equivalents/paid hour	7.93	7.04	6.34
Meal equivalents/FTE	1,371	1,219	1,097

Figure 11E.
Daily Sales Analysis

Date	Period*	Sales	No. of customers	Average check	Labor cost					
					Management	Preparation	Service	Sanitation	Total	
Jan. 1	Breakfast Lunch Dinner									
Jan. 2										
Jan. 31										
Total										

*May include a.m. and p.m. coffee breaks and catering functions.

Figure 11F.
Daily Sales (Menu) Record

Date	Period	Description	Number served	Food cost	Total sales
Jan. 4	Breakfast	Scrambled eggs Pancakes Bacon Oatmeal			
	Lunch	Chili Hamburger Beef tips/noodles Roast turkey Broiled haddock			
	Dinner	Baked chicken Roast beef Liver w/onions			

CHAPTER 12
VENDING MACHINES

In hospitals, as in many areas with a potential to sell food or beverages 24 hours a day, vending machines are a common sight. Still uncommon is the ownership of vending machines by hospitals and the operation of those machines by the food service department. If there is a potential to sell more food and beverages than are currently being sold, because of potential customers during hours when the cafeteria is not open or because certain items could be sold but display space in the cafeteria is not available, then there is a potential for vending machines. If vending machines are used but are operated under contract by an outside contractor, there is a potential for the contract to be cancelled, the machines to be purchased and operated internally, and the profit that formerly went to the outside contractor to be retained by the hospital.

The food service administrator manages an operation that buys, stores, prepares, and serves food. Equipment, employees, nonfood supplies, and money are managed in the provision of the food. Vending machine operation is merely an extension of these components from traditional, manual food service to automatic food service.

The nine types of vending machines of most interest to the hospital vending operator are hot beverage; window-front merchandiser; candy, cookie, and cracker; cup cold beverage; canned or bottled cold beverage; all-purpose food; canned juice and milk; pastry; and ice cream.

There are many different manufacturers of vending machines, and machines vary in their versatility. It is not unusual to vend juice, milk, pastry, sandwiches, and other items from a single machine, although at least three different types of machines are designed to vend one or more of those items specifically. Meetings with sales people who represent the various manufacturers will lead to the selection of the most appropriate vending machines for a specific hospital. One possible source of loaner machines is through soda vendors. Bottlers and syrup vendors that serve a hospital's geographic area should be contacted and requested to supply either a canned or bottled cold beverage machine or cup cold beverage machine in exchange for exclusive use of the vendor's product in the machine. This, of course, eliminates the capital expense to the hospital while providing the mechanism to vend a very popular and profitable product.

The initial investment required to start up a vending operation depends greatly on the machines selected. Prices range, generally, from just under $2,000 for a simple machine, such as a hot beverage vendor, to over $4,000 for a more complicated machine, such as a window-front merchandiser. Discounts of up to 25% may be available when more than one machine is purchased, depending on the policies of the selected manufacturer and distributor. The depreciable life of most vending machines is seven years.

The actual profit or loss, net return, and pay-out period for a vending operation will depend on the volume of business and the pricing of the vended products. An example follows of the effect on one hospital of removal of an outside vending contractor, purchase of vending machines, and operation of those machines by the food service department.

The hospital has a cafeteria that operates from 6:30 a.m. to 7:00 p.m. every day and a coffee shop that is open from 9:00 a.m. to 4:00 p.m. every day except Sunday. The vending machines were located in a low-traffic, service-elevator lobby, so they produced less than their potential volume of sales. In this case vending was needed primarily to make food and beverage available from 7:00 p.m. to 6:30 a.m., when no other service was available. The outside contractor had operated vending machines for one and a half years in the hospital but had returned minimal commission although the contract called for a rebate of 20% of sales. The outside contractor operated a canned cold beverage machine, a hot beverage machine, and a candy machine. It also rented a window-front merchandiser for $100 per month to the food service department, which operated it. The food service administrator determined that a hot beverage machine, a candy and snack machine, and a sandwich machine could be purchased for $4,700 and that these machines, combined with a canned cold beverage machine supplied by a major soda bottler in exchange for exclusive use of the bottler's product in the machine, would meet the hospital's vending needs. The profile of the initial investment justification was:

Preliminary Assumptions

$4,700	Capital investment, 7-year life

Estimated Operating Statement, Monthly

$1,076	Sales
	Operating expenses
$ 430	Food and supplies at 40%
$ 420	Labor at 39%
$ 56	Depreciation ($4,700 ÷ 84 months)
$ 906	Total operating expenses
$ 170	Net profit

Average Rate of Return

$$\frac{\$170 \text{ (monthly net profit)} \times 12 \text{ months}}{\$4,700 \text{ capital investment}} = 43.4\%$$

Payback Period

$$\frac{\$4,700 \text{ capital investment}}{\$170 \text{ (monthly net profit)} \times 12 \text{ months}} = 2.3 \text{ years}$$

After the vending machines had been in operation for one year, it was determined that the net profit averaged $255.23 per month, not $170 per month, changing the average rate of return to 65.2% and the payback period to 1.53 years.

To break even on the above capital expenditure, which was depreciated at $56 per month, required sales of $230.51 per month. This was calculated on the basis of a food and supply cost of 40% of sales, other expenses such as repairs and licensing of 1% of sales, and labor of 10% of sales. However, labor was calculated as a fixed cost up to $80 per month, as that level was considered necessary to ensure quality, freshness, and availability of the products to be vended. Thus:

40% sales + 1% sales + $56 depreciation + $80 labor = 100% sales
   to break even
41% sales + $136 = sales
$136 = 59% sales
$136 ÷ 59% = sales
$230.51 = sales/month to break even

Vending machine operation lends itself very readily to tight controls. As many of the products vended are prepackaged in wrappers, bags, cans, or bottles, portion control techniques need be exercised only on freshly made products such as sandwiches, salads, and entrees if those items are offered. Cash controls are simplified as there is no cashier at the point of sale, and money is handled by workers only at the time the locked cash box is counted. The perpetual inventory format is usually applicable, because all but fresh food can be kept in its own storeroom, which needs to be accessible only to a service worker and management. Fresh foods can be requisitioned from the cafeteria or patient area as needed, requiring no separate inventory. A requisition form such as the one illustrated in figure 5C, Resale Food Requisition, can be used for the requisition and cost transfer reference between vending and the area that produces the freshly made food items. Appropriate items are listed in the designated column of the form.

Figure 12A illustrates a sample storeroom inventory form. The column headings show that space is provided next to each item to enter the opening inventory, items placed into or taken out of inventory, a running balance, the ending inventory, total of items used, unit cost, and the extended cost of all the items used. Every item recorded as withdrawn from the inventory must appear in an "Add" column of a control sheet (see figure 12B).

Figure 12B illustrates a control sheet for one machine, in this case a snack vendor. Each type of machine used would have a similar form but with items listed appropriate to that type. The control sheet is kept in the vending machine for one accounting period—one week, four weeks, or a month—and acts as an individual inventory for that machine. Space is provided for the beginning inventory, additions to the machine's inventory, removals from the inventory, the ending inventory, the number of items sold ("Beginning Inventory" plus "Total In" minus "Total Out"), the price charged for each item, and a sales column ("Number Sold" times "Price"). Every item that appears in an "Add" column comes from the storeroom and appears in an "Out" column on the storeroom inventory or comes from the cafeteria or patient area and appears on a requisition sent to that area. Space on the vending control sheet is also provided for recording readings on the transaction meter that counts the number of times the machine vends an item and a space for reconciliation of sales with cash collected.

In practice the vending storeroom inventory, vending control sheet, and requisition are used in this way:

1. At the beginning of the accounting period, a member of management inventories the vending storeroom and records the count of each item in the "Beginning Inventory" column of the vending storeroom inventory (figure 12A). The top of the column is initialed and dated by the inventory taker. That person then goes to each vending machine and records the inventory of each item in the machine in the "Beginning Inventory" column of that machine's vending control sheet (figure 12B). The inventory taker initials and dates the top of the column, records the beginning date of the accounting period, and records the reading on the machine's transaction meter next to "Meter Beginning" (figure 12B). It should be noted that the beginning count of a new accounting period is also used as an ending count for the previous accounting period.

2. As vending items are purchased during the accounting period, they are entered into an "In" column of the vending storeroom inventory, the "Balance" column is increased by the number of items purchased, and the worker placing the items into inventory dates and initials the top of the column in which the entry is made.

3. As items are taken from the storeroom for placement in a vending machine, the vending service worker records the items that are removed from the storeroom in the "Out" column of the vending storeroom inventory, decreases the "Balance" column accordingly, and dates and initials the top of the column.

4. Upon delivery of the items to the vending machine, the service worker records the items placed in the machine in the "Add" column and dates and initials the top of the column.

5. For items placed in a vending machine but not kept in the vending storeroom, the service worker issues a requisition listing the items needed. Those items are entered into the machine as indicated in step 4, above.

6. Cash is collected from each machine at appropriate intervals during the accounting period. The person who collects the cash should be a member of management, definitely not the service worker, and preferably not the person responsible for reconciling the vending account. Deposits should be made separately for each collection of money from each machine, or the deposits may be consolidated, but the money collected from each machine should be recorded separately on standard columnar accounting forms.

7. The "Test" line is provided on the vending control sheet (figure 12B) in the event a machine malfunctions and test vends must be made to ascertain correction of the malfunction. A free vend switch is used to make the machine vend without placing money in it. Although the item(s) vended should be returned to the machine by the tester, the transaction meter will record a transaction for every free vend. Therefore, tests must be recorded so that they can be subtracted from meter transactions at the time of reconciliation and actual cash transactions can be determined.

8. At the end of the accounting period, inventories are taken as outlined

in step 1 but, of course, using "Ending" inventory columns, dates, and meter readings on the vending control sheet. The next period's beginning information should be recorded at the same time.

9. All inventories, requisitions, control sheets, and records of deposit should be submitted to a member of management, probably the food service administrator, at the end of the accounting period.

The information submitted is generated by three different people: the service worker, the inventory taker, and the cash handler. This makes collusion less likely because of the number of people involved. Calculation of extensions may be delegated, but it is now up to one worker to reconcile the period's vending operation as recorded by these three individuals as well as by each machine's meter. The procedure is as follows:

1. The inventories, control sheets, and requisitions should be extended to determine the value of products used. On the inventory form, check to be sure that the "Beginning Inventory" plus "In" minus "Out" equals "Ending Inventory." On the control form the "Beginning Inventory" plus "Add" minus ("Removals" plus "Ending Inventory") equals "Number Sold." Every entry in an "Out" column of the inventory should match entries in the "Add" columns of control forms on the date the inventory withdrawal was made. Every item requisitioned should appear as an "Add" on the control sheets.

2. The extended sales value of each item listed on each control sheet should be totaled to arrive at the value of sales for each machine according to the information supplied by the service worker and the inventory taker.

3. The total deposits made for each machine should be entered on the "Cash Deposit" line of each control sheet indicating the value of sales according to the information supplied by the cash handler. This should equal total sales as determined in step 2. Any difference is recorded as "Over/Short" and is subject to further investigation.

4. The number of tests recorded is subtracted from the difference between the beginning and ending meter readings to show the number of cash transactions recorded by each machine. This figure should equal the total of the "Number Sold" column of each machine. When only one price is charged for all products vended by a machine, the net meter reading can be multiplied by that selling price to arrive at a total value of sales from a third source.

5. The food and supply cost for each machine can be determined in either of two ways. One, by extending the number of each item sold, as recorded on the control sheet, by the cost of the item and then totaling the costs of all items on the control sheet, the total food and supply cost for each machine is determined on an accrual basis. Two, by taking the costs determined on the requisitions and inventory forms, and applying them against each machine according to its receipt of each item, the cost is determined on a cash basis. Either method is acceptable, although the accrual basis is a bit tighter because it reflects inventory variances.

6. With transaction counts, sales volume, and food and supply cost information at hand, the vending report (see figure 12C) can be prepared. Every machine should be listed in the left column, with the information for each machine supplied to the right. The figure for the "Customers"

column comes from the "Net Meter" reading on the vending control sheet. The "Sales" column reflects the cash deposit made for each machine during the period. The figure for the "Cost" column is as determined in step 5, above. The "Gain (Loss)" figure is the difference between "Sales" and "Cost." From this gross figure labor cost, repairs, license fees, and any other expenses should be subtracted to arrive at the "Net Operating Gain (Loss)" for the period. Figure 12C illustrates a report for an operation with four machines of different types. Additional types of machines could be listed or additional machines of a type could be listed with some predetermined identification such as numbers or locations, for example, "Soda-1st floor," "Soda-3rd floor."

Most vending machines require product rotation by their design. It is unlikely that spoilage would ever be a concern in any machine except a fresh food vendor. Reasonable guidelines should be set up and maintained for vending fresh foods. Because machines that vend fresh foods are refrigerated, fruits remain salable through their normal refrigerator life, and yogurt and milk products are safe through their normal sale-date codes. Freshly made products such as sandwiches, salads, entrees, and baked goods have a more limited life. It should be realized that once an item is placed in a refrigerated machine it will taste refrigerated, not fresh, although some hot items can be reconstituted reasonably well in a microwave oven, a common accessory in a vending area. Standards for fresh foods and their rotation must be established by the individual location. A common standard is anywhere from one to three days in the machine before removal if not sold. An identification sticker on this type of item, as is required by law in some states, is a good place to mark an expiration code.

Pricing vended food is also very much up to the individual operation. Because the labor cost is relatively low for hospital self-operated vending compared to patient service, cafeteria operation, or an outside contractor, it would be possible to price vended food lower than cafeteria prices and still achieve the same financial objectives as in the cafeteria. Also, because vending, unless placed in a restricted-access area, is available to the public as well as to employees, there is justification for charging higher, more profitable prices. The pricing policy decided on should reflect the hospital's philosophy on vending and should be based on the principles presented in chapter 5, Menu Pricing.

The vending business fits very well into the operation of the food service department. As previously mentioned, it is merely an extension of services and operations that the department experiences in providing manual services. With minimal training, almost any food service employee can be trained to service a vending machine on a full-time or part-time basis, depending on the size of the vending operation. Fresh foods should be selected from those being produced in either the cafeteria or the patient area, and prepackaged products need only be purchased, stored, and put in machines in their as purchased form. If the hospital is going to provide vending services, it is in the best interest of the institution to have the food service department manage them.

Figure 12A.
Vending Storeroom Inventory

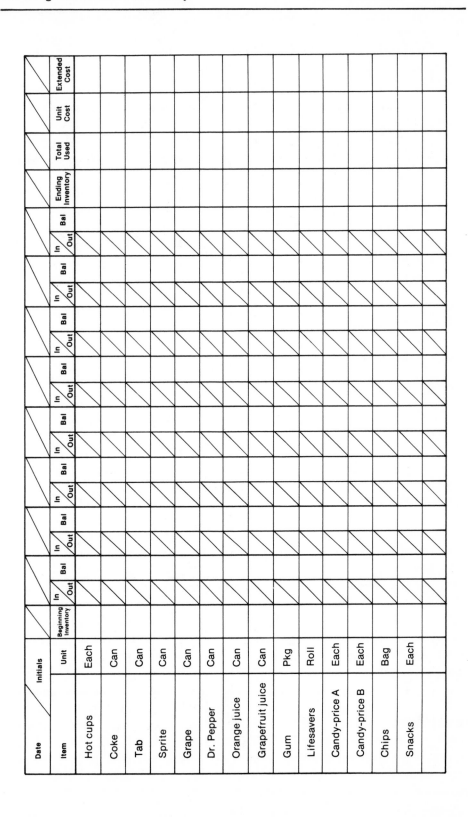

Figure 12B.
Vending Control Sheet

Item	Beginning inventory	Add	Add	Add	Add	Add	Add	Add	Add	Add	Add	Add	Add	Total in	Removed	Removed	Ending inventory	Total out	Number sold	Price	Sales
Candy																					
Gum																					
Lifesavers																					
Snacks																					
Chips																					
Cakes																					
Tests																					

Date Beginning _____
Ending _____

Snack

Cash audit _____

Initials _____
Date _____

Meter ending _____
Meter beginning _____
Meter sales _____

Meter sales _____
Tests _____
Net meter _____

Total sales $ _____
Cash deposit $ _____
Over / short $ _____

Figure 12C.
Vending Report

	Customers	Sales	Cost	Gain (loss)
Month_____				
Year _____				
Hot beverage				
Soda				
Sandwich				
Snack				
Total				
Less: Labor ---				
Other ---				
Net operating gain (loss)				

Net operating gain (loss) year to date:

CHAPTER 13
MERCHANDISING AND MARKETING

MERCHANDISING

The following three-step approach to cultivating an image, satisfying patrons, and increasing sales is suggested by Sill (ref. 13):

1. *Positioning.* To develop an understanding of the competitive situation, the food service administrator should first analyze the market place—defining the make-up of the total market, current customers, and the target market—and put the results of the analysis in writing. After examining all the elements of the marketing unit as they relate to the cafeteria, the food service administrator should define his or her attitudes, the physical shape of the plant, and the standards of performance that in turn shape the dining experience and create, in the customer's mind, an image of the cafeteria.

2. *Cafeteria Personality.* Customers personalize a restaurant, forming an image of it based not only on the type and quality of the food but on many intangibles as well. The owner can guide the development of this image, imbuing his restaurant with a distinctive personality. Wenzel (ref. 14), a well-known restaurant consultant, advises owners that there should be "a smile on the face of the cashier when (the guest comes) in, and on the waitress when she approaches, and on the busboy when he helps clear the table. These employees must be taught this. They won't do it if the owner doesn't set the example. . . . And, obviously, they must be rewarded to show that you appreciate their cooperation." Sill points out that the personality of the restaurant should also be evident in its physical features.

3. *Merchandising Services.* Sill recommends that by methodically going through each step—questioning motives, defining objectives, establishing standards, and creating atmosphere—the owner has essentially developed the underlying merchandising strategy for his or her restaurant. All that remains is the implementation of merchandising techniques and tactics.

Actually, in the hospital cafeteria point-of-sale merchandising—the things that can be done to promote the sale of food once the customer is in the door—will increase sales and profitability. There are certain basic requirements that must be met, or the best merchandising campaign will be negated:

- The physical appearance of the cafeteria must be clean, orderly, and pleasant. It is not necessary to be fancy or new, but it must be a comfortable place where the customer can feel relaxed while purchasing food and services.

- The food must be good. It must look good, smell good, and taste good or the most attractive garnishes available will be wasted.
- The third required ingredient is the staff. The cafeteria employees should be well trained, pleasant, clean people who enjoy serving the customers.

With the basics taken care of, a merchandising program can be started by trying the following:

- Garnish every food item tastefully. Be more imaginative than sticking parsley or whipped topping on everything. Most fruits and vegetables can be cut or sliced into attractive garnishes. Raisins, nuts, shredded coconut, granola, croutons, dry gelatin, and citrus fruits are particularly useful as garnishes.
- Have a steam-table plan for every menu. Mix the colors of the food items so that they provide a pleasing contrast to one another.
- Have dessert and salad area plans. Again, mix the colors. Separate coleslaw, potato salad, and cottage cheese from each other with more colorful salads. Make sure these areas are neat. Whether items are set out in straight rows, diagonals, or a checkerboard, make sure the set-up is adhered to.
- Use bulk displays. Whole cakes and pies are great dessert area decorations. Baskets of fruit look better than individual pieces of fruits on plates. Bowls of bulk salads from which portions are dished as needed can be displayed on the salad counter just behind the individual portions of that item.
- Carve or slice roasts to order right on the serving line. Be sure to have plenty ready, as this really sells meat.
- Train all food service employees to use the same greeting. "May I serve you?" sounds better than "Next." Make sure that food servers and cashiers say "Thank you" to each customer.
- Train food servers to promote add-on sales. If a customer orders a hamburger, the server should not wait for the customer to ask for french fries but should immediately say, "Would you like french fries with your hamburger?" All customers should be asked which vegetables they would like and whether they would like a cup or a bowl of today's soup.
- Hold preservice meetings in the serving area just prior to opening. These meetings should include taste-testing by the employees who will serve the food so that they will know they are serving good food, and an explanation of each item by a cook or supervisor so the server can describe any item to an unsure customer. This is also a good time to review portion control, showing examples with each item to be served.
- Offer larger portions at higher prices. If a 12-oz soft drink is the standard portion, offer a 16-oz cup at a higher price. It will increase sales without increasing prices of the standard portion. This concept is discussed in detail in chapter 5.
- Feature a special item of the day. Make it something different and offer a copy of the recipe, reduced for home use. Try this idea in all areas— hot food, salads, desserts, and sandwiches.

The preceding ideas are presented as a good beginning to a merchandising program. The reason for using them and for all merchandising ideas is that merchandising makes the customer want to buy the items merchandised, buy more of them, and buy them more often.

MARKETING

The primary business of every business is to stay in business, and to do that you have to get and keep customers. To accomplish this objective, you have to sell a product and/or service that is needed or desired by a certain number of customers.

Actually, all of us constantly sell something, even if only our skills and personalities. As a rule, we sell eagerly but we buy suspiciously. As customers, our first reaction to a sale situation is caution or perhaps sometimes fear: Are we being "sold a bill of goods?"

For one thing, the seller usually knows more about the defects or limitations of a product and/or a service than the buyer. The seller is an expert, the buyer at best is only a well informed amateur. The seller can seldom know everything the buyer really requires, and even less of what he or she really wants.

In fact, the seller-buyer relationship is a transaction in which each side gets something it wants that the other side has in its possession. In this selling-buying situation, if the seller digs deeply enough to discover the real needs and wants of the buyer, the seller can create and provide the desired product and/or service. The process of doing this kind of digging and the action that follows is called *marketing*. Specifically, marketing means that the seller attempts to find out what the customer's needs and wants are and tries to create or modify an existing product and/or service so that the customer will really prefer it over all its competitors. An example of accomplishing an effective marketing survey in the hospital food service cafeteria is outlined in chapter 16.

However, for the purpose of this chapter, marketing is actually an aggregate of functions used to move goods from the producer to the consumer. The term *marketing* is used here as an umbrella term under which to offer a few ideas that will attract the customer to the cafeteria so that the ongoing merchandising program will keep him coming back. Also, marketing is used to sell a special idea or item. Some approaches to hospital cafeteria marketing are as follows:

- Publish the menu. Do this at least a week in advance and distribute it so that everyone who might be attracted as a customer will see it.
- Hold special events, advertise them in advance, and use decorations, music, costumes—everything available—to create the atmosphere. Nationality days, ethnic days, and holidays are popular special events. Make-your-own-sundae (or whatever), cheesecake day, and strawberry festivals are all variations of featuring a single item and are very popular.
- Promote take-home sales. As long as food is produced that is properly priced, it is advantageous to sell as much as possible.
- Offer a come-on to build sales during slow periods. Free popcorn in the

afternoon doesn't cost much but does increase beverage sales during a slow period.

- Offer special prices during off hours. A 10% discount on breakfast during the slowest half hour or hour will bring in additional customers and cover the food cost while helping to meet the labor cost.
- Follow the trends or set them. If salad bars and frozen yogurt are popular, sell them. Find out what people want to buy, tell them that they can buy it in the hospital cafeteria, then sell it to them profitably.

Part B of this publication studies marketing for the hospital cafeteria in depth. Marketing is mentioned in this chapter to emphasize its place as a normal part of the daily routine of the food service administrator. The surveys and other techniques discussed in part B will not be performed in their entirety on a daily basis, for obvious reasons. However, marketing and merchandising are as important to the proper management of the hospital cafeteria as are menu planning, establishment of standards, or any other aspect of management discussed in part A.

Part B. Audit and Marketing Techniques

CHAPTER 14
INTRODUCTION TO PART B

Hospital cafeterias have seen major changes in emphasis during the past ten years. Operations that were once an afterthought in hospital planning have begun to have their own dedicated space. Hospital cafeterias are no longer a place to use up overproduction, but rather a place to offer a food service program to sophisticated and demanding customers. Many hospital cafeterias are now staffed by professional managers and must now compete for business with fast-food shops and restaurants.

Along with this updating of philosophy and outlook are increased demands to meet the needs of the following different factions simultaneously:

- Hospital administrators see the cafeteria as an employee benefit, a cost to the institution in space and dollars, and a problem if it is not being run well.
- Employees see the cafeteria as a low-cost alternative to bringing their lunch from home and as a place to meet their co-workers away from the pressures of the job.
- Patients see the cafeteria as a convenience for their visitors and for themselves when they return as an outpatient.
- Third-party payers see the cafeteria as a nonpatient expense requiring strict cost containment efforts.
- Food service administrators see the cafeteria as a substantial portion of their work, involving the feeding of five or six times the number of people fed in the patient area.

How does one meet all of these needs simultaneously? A cafeteria will meet these needs equitably if it offers a high-quality program with variety and choice, is efficiently managed, and breaks even or makes a contribution toward indirect costs. The question, then, seems to be: "Can I offer a high-quality operation with variety and choice that does not cost the hospital or patients any money?"

The high-quality, choice, and variety are not too difficult to achieve. Food service administrators ask their customers what they want and then give it to them. If this is done with a high-quality program at a reasonable price, success is imminent.

The difficulty often lies in doing this and in making a few dollars, or at least breaking even, at the same time.

The competition does it, though, and a hospital cafeteria can too. Fast-food shops, restaurants, and delis are in the same business—the food service business. If they are still open after a year, they are probably making money and satisfying their customers.

They do this by planning. They collect data and make informed decisions about how to be in business and stay in business. The cafeteria audit and marketing technique is a planning process that can be used in a hospital cafeteria operation. It is simple, straightforward, adaptable to most operations, and a proven success.

Part B provides a systematic approach for food service administrators to evaluate, analyze, and plan action for their cafeteria operations. Part B consists of a self-audit process with many different parts so that food service administrators can customize their study to fit their own operations.

Chapters 15-22 consist of eight mini-studies in the areas of the facility, the customer, sales volume and average check, food cost, menu, what customers are buying, the competition, and break-even. These eight mini-studies are the most important part of the audit and take the most time.

Chapters 23 and 24 deal with how to work on difficulties or opportunities that may have been identified in the mini-studies. Most of these ideas are general in nature to allow for individual planning to fit a particular hospital cafeteria. Chapter 25 deals with developing an operating strategy and setting goals and objectives. Chapter 26 deals with planning and provides an action planning process with examples.

CHAPTER 15
OPERATIONS CHECKLIST

There are eight areas in the operations checklist. Within each area, there are a number of self-evaluation questions to be answered. These questions are planned to provide an opportunity for food service administrators to think about their operation from their customers' viewpoint. After each question has been reviewed, some notes should be made regarding items that may need some improvements, from either the administrator's or the customers' viewpoint. A final list of items to work on should be saved for later use.

Some food service administrators have found it helpful to have a hospital administrator or another person not involved in the direct management of the cafeteria assist in this review. Often, the differing viewpoints provide startling results.

1. *Physical layout*
    a. Is the cafeteria accessible to all customers?
    b. Are the entrances and exits clearly marked?
    c. Are tray, silverware, and napkin locations easily identified?
    d. Is line placement logical from a customer's standpoint? Does it promote a free flow of customers?
    e. Are the different functional areas clearly identified?
    f. Are there any production bottlenecks or crossing patterns that would inhibit customer movement?
    g. Are there enough cash registers to handle peak flow?
    h. Are there tray stands or slides at all locations where customers may need to rest their tray?
    i. Does the lighting effectively highlight food selections, make sign reading easy, and allow for easy movement through the area?
2. *Customer communications*
    a. Are the hours of operation posted in an accessible location?
    b. Are the menu boards clean, neat, readable, and organized?
    c. Are most food selections labeled and priced?
    d. Are the "Specials of the Day" posted and explained?
    e. Are there directional signs to help customers move through the serving area?
    f. Is there a suggestion box for customer input?
    g. Are smoking and nonsmoking areas clearly marked?
3. *Product quality and quantity*
    a. Are the products available the ones that you decided should be there?

    b. Are they the ones that customers are asking for?
    c. Are the portions the same as the ones you base your pricing on?
    d. Do the products look the way you want them to look?
    e. Are all the portions for the same product the same size and quality?
    f. Is there a portion control list in the cafeteria?
 4. *Pricing*
    a. Are all items clearly priced?
    b. Are items that are value-priced clearly marked as specials?
    c. Is there a daily special that is a good deal for customers? Do customers know it's a good deal—what and how much?
    d. Are larger items a better value than multiples of smaller items?
 5. *Food displays*
    a. Are food displays orderly? Do they reflect a high-quality image?
    b. Does the line reflect the statement that people eat with their eyes? Does the presentation make customers want to try something new?
    c. Does the line feature the items that you want to sell the most?
    d. Is the display designed to affect customers' buying patterns?
    e. Are items refilled before they run out?
    f. Are you taking maximum advantage of self-service items? Are those items that are self-service, truly self-service?
 6. *Sanitation*
    a. Are the service and dining areas clean and neat?
    b. Are there appropriate waste containers for disposables?
    c. Is the area picked up on a regular basis?
    d. Is the tray-return area clearly marked?
    e. Are ashtrays available in the smoking section?
 7. *Employees*
    a. Are employees clean and neat in appearance?
    b. Do they have the proper uniform on?
    c. Are they wearing name tags?
    d. Do they demonstrate a "may I help you" attitude?
    e. Are they customer-aware? Do they foresee customer needs?
    f. Is the cashier courteous?
    g. Are there sufficient employees to meet customer needs? Are there too few or too many?
    h. Is the manager or supervisor visible and available to promote high-quality service?
 8. *Dining area*
    a. Which of these words best define the dining area: congenial, quiet, noisy, busy, empty, clean, messy, comfortable, sterile, inviting?
    b. Are the sizes, number, and variety of tables sufficient to meet customer needs?
    c. Is the temperature, ventilation, and lighting appropriate to the environment you want your customers to eat in?
    d. Are there private spots for quiet moments or personal discussions?
    e. What type of tray-bussing is being used? Does it work?

After working through this checklist, food service administrators should list the items that they want to work on at a later date. If any solutions have been thought of, those should also be noted at this time.

CHAPTER 16
MARKET SURVEY
AND SEGMENTATION STUDY

In this chapter, the desired end result is a better understanding of customers and of the hospital cafeteria's present ability to meet their needs. These are some questions that the food service administrator should be able to answer:

1. Who are the customers?
2. How many are in the potential market of this cafeteria?
3. What are their needs?
4. How much do they eat?
5. How often do they use this facility?
6. When do they use this facility?
7. How much do they spend?
8. Who is not being served and what steps can be taken to meet those needs?

The answers to these questions will be summarized on the Market Survey and Segmentation Study (figure 16A).

The hospital food service administrator is probably the best resource to begin answering question number one. Some quick responses here might be these: physicians, nurses, interns, residents, administrators, secretaries, office staff, service staff (housekeeping, laundry, food service), visitors, and outpatients. There may be some other markets that may be important to consider— outside contractors, students, and volunteers are often missed. Every hospital has its own distinct market. Cashiers, supervisors, the administrator, and possibly the security staff can help determine whether anyone has been missed.

Once the list is completed, it should be consolidated by buying pattern. This is a judgment call for the food service administrator. It is better to isolate a group and do a little more work than to consolidate to the point where the information is not totally valid. Each market has very distinct buying patterns that relate to its life style, and the successful food service administrator attempts to satisfy as many of these patterns as possible. Two groups that usually can be consolidated are physicians and house staff (residents). Most of the others have distinctly different buying patterns.

The next step is to list each group separately on the Market Survey and Segmentation Study (form 16A), column 1.

Market potential (column 4) will take a bit of research. The number needed here is the total number of persons in a market segment on a daily basis. The size of groups such as nurses, house staff, service staff, administrators, and others on the hospital payroll can be obtained through the personnel office. If the information is available, an approximate breakdown by shift should be determined, because buying patterns usually vary by the time of day. The number of outpatients can be determined through outpatient admitting, volunteers through the volunteer office, and students through medical education. Other segments may be more difficult. Sometimes, members of a group must be asked where the information can be gathered. Otherwise, an educated estimate will have to be used. The average number of persons in each segment should be entered on a daily basis (Monday through Friday) in column 4.

Once the different segments of the market and the potential size of each have been determined, the food service administrator should begin to focus on each segment's needs and the degree to which those needs are being met. There are two techniques to use to gather this information.

The first is called a focus group. In this process the hospital food service administrator should sit down and discuss with two to six representatives of a market segment, for example, nurses or housekeeping staff, their needs and expectations with regard to the cafeteria operation. This discussion should be as informal as possible. It is important, however, to be specific and to have a list of questions planned in advance. One good approach is to explain what the focus group is and to offer to buy the coffee. This is a good ice breaker. Start with general questions and gradually become more specific. Some sample questions might include:

- What are your expectations of the cafeteria?
- Are we meeting your needs? If not, what should be done differently?
- How often do you use the facility?

This process is rather time-consuming and should be limited to one or two focus group meetings per market segment, with each meeting lasting not more than 15 minutes. There are some instances where focus grouping may not be possible.

The key element in focus grouping is to begin determining an overview of customers' reactions to the operation. This overview will provide the basis for the second step of information gathering, the survey. Many of the questions in the survey should attempt to verify the information discovered in the focus groups.

The survey will be able to deal with more specific questions and with more people, and it will provide the information needed to complete the market needs/preferences portion of the study.

The survey should be kept as short as possible while still requesting all the needed information. The maximum length should be two typed pages. The questions should address those issues raised in the focus groups as well as the answers to those questions asked at the beginning of this chapter.

Each survey will be different because each addresses a different market situation. Two samples, figures 16B and 16C, are included to offer some guidance. It is important to include questions that will help isolate segments and their individual needs. As many copies of the survey should be sent out as can be tabulated. The more returns received, the better the understanding of customers' needs.

Once the survey results are returned, the data should be tabulated and summarized. This information should be broken down by market segment. Then the market need/preferences section (column 2) of the Market Survey and Segmentation Study can be completed.

To determine the number for column 3, "Currently Being Served," a tally sheet broken down by predetermined segments should be developed. Using the tally sheet, the cashier can record the segment a customer is in after each transaction. This task is usually quite easy because most hospital personnel wear name tags. The tally should be as accurate as possible without offending customers. During busy periods an extra person may have to be put on the tally process.

This process should be done for two to three days. At the end of the time allotted, a daily average for each segment should be computed and entered in column 3.

Column 4 minus column 3 equals column 5, the growth potential for each segment. These are the potential customers to whom some marketing efforts should be directed. These efforts should include those market needs and preferences listed in column 2.

Column 6, "Changes/Opportunities Indicated," is for notes regarding efforts necessary to make the operation more customer-oriented and, it is hoped, more profitable. The following are some ideas:

- Add items in column 2 that you are not selling at present
- Increase the use of high preference items
- Eliminate items not frequently requested
- Add items that will create growth in segments not heavily saturated (column 5)
- Add items that customers indicated they go to the competition for

The final step (column 7) is to rank the different segments by greatest potential for increased business. This ranking will be helpful in developing an action plan at the end of the audit.

Figure 16A.
Market Survey and Segmentation Study

Market Segment 1	Market Need/Preferences 2	Currently Being Served (Daily) 3	Market Potential (Daily) 4	Growth Potential (Daily) 5	Changes/Opportunities Indicated 6	Priority Rank 7
NURSING DAY SHIFT 7:00 a.m. – 3:30 p.m.	Diet items Salad bar Like vegetarian items Dislike entrees – too expensive Average uses per week: Lunch 4x Break 6x	312	525	213	1. Develop salad bar and direct promotional activity at nurses. 2. There is currently a low market penetration. 3. Add more low cost vegetarian items. 4. Begin a diet plate program featuring calorie and nutrient information.	1
SERVICE EMPLOYEES	Soup and sandwich are a priority. They do not utilize entrees very often. Several mentioned their preference for our home-made muffins. Many bring lunch from home but buy beverage and snack in cafeteria. Average uses per week: Lunch 4X Break 5X	391	473	82	1. Develop a sandwich program of items not available at home. For example: hot ham and cheese, pastrami. 2. Introduce new "Souper" sandwich with a soup and sandwich combination.	2

Figure 16B.
Sample Survey 1

Dear Customer:

   As part of our annual review of nonpatient food services, we are undertaking a study of cafeteria operations to determine how well we are meeting your needs. We would appreciate it if you would fill out this survey to assist us in this process.

   Please check or fill in each response as it applies to you.

1. The name that best describes my position at the Medical Center is:

   ___ Physician   ___ Department head

   ___ Nurse   ___ Service staff (laundry, food services, housekeeping)

   ___ Administrator   ___ Outpatient

   ___ Office staff   ___ Visitor

2. On the average how may times do you use the cafeteria *each week*?

   Full meal ___ times

   Snack/break ___ times

3. What time of day do you use the facility?

   Full meal ___

   Snack/break ___

4. How much do you normally spend for one meal and/or one break?

   Full meal ___

   Snack/break ___

5. What is the item or service that we provide that you like best?

   _____

   _____

   What is the item or service that you like least?

   _____

   _____

6. Are our employees helpful and attentive to your needs?

   ___ Always   ___ Usually   ___ Sometimes   ___ Not very often

7. If you could add 3 menu items to the menu, what would they be and how much should they cost?

ITEM	COST
1. _____	_____
2. _____	_____
3. _____	_____

8. Where do you go as an alternative to the cafeteria?

   _____   _____

   What does that operation do that attracts you there?

   _____   _____

Thanks for your help. Please return survey to the box provided.

Date _____   Food Service Department
                             XYZ Medical Center

Figure 16C.
Sample Survey 2

WE NEED YOUR HELP . . . . . .
So that we may better serve you, we need your answers to the following questions.
We will use this information in planning our program to meet our customer needs.

1. With what part of the hospital are you associated?
   Physician ____ Nurse ____ Administrator ____ Service Staff ____ Office Staff ____ Other (specify) _____

2. How often do you visit the cafeteria?
   Once a week ____ . Twice a week ____ . . 3 or more times a week ____ . Every day ____ .
   More than once a day ____ .

3. On what day(s) of the week do you use the cafeteria facilities?
   Monday ____ Tuesday ____ Wednesday ____ Thursday ____ Friday ____ Saturday ____ Sunday ____

4. What time(s) of the day do you usually visit the cafeteria?
   6:30-10:00 ____ 10:00-12:00 ____ 12:00-2:00 ____ 2:00-5:00 ____ 5:00-7:00 ____ Other (specify) _____

5. Why do you choose the cafeteria? (Check more than one if necessary).
   Food ____ Prices ____ Meet friends ____ Convenience ____ Other (specify) _____

6. What do you usually purchase?
   Sandwich ____ Grill items ____ Salad Bar ____ Coffee "and" ____ Breakfast ____
   Beverages ____ Dessert ____ Soup or Chowder ____

7. How much do you usually spend?
   25¢ or less ____ 25¢ to 50¢ ____ 50¢ to $1.00 ____ $1.00 to $1.50 ____ $1.50 or more ____

8. What is your favorite item in the cafeteria?

9. What is your least favorite thing?
   What would you like to see added to the menu?
   At what price range?

10. What is another fast-food shop that you like?
    What do they do that you would like us to do?

Date _____

THANK YOU.
Food Service Department
XYZ Medical Center

CHAPTER 17
CASH REGISTER SALES ANALYSIS

The Cash Register Sales Analysis (figure 17A) is designed to assist the food service administrator in determining:
- Average check
- Sales per hour
- Sales per paid hour
- Customers served per paid hour

This process is meaningful not only as part of the overall audit but also on a continuing basis as a determiner of an operation's productivity.

The average check figure will be used later on in the audit to determine potential sales for underutilized markets. For purposes of the audit, the cashier should complete one Cash Register Sales Analysis each day for one week. At the end of a week, a weekly composite should be completed. The composite will be used in later calculations.

To complete the Cash Register Sales Analysis, the food service administrator should:

1. Have the cashier take an hourly register reading (column A) and hourly customer count (column C). If there is more than one cash register, each cashier should complete the hourly reading and customer count, with the food service administrator compiling the information into a single composite before going to step 2.

2. Complete column B by subtracting the previous hour's sales from the current hour's sales to give net sales for the current hour. For example, the 9:00 a.m. reading should be subtracted from the 10:00 a.m. reading to give hourly sales from 9:00 to 10:00 a.m. This should be done for each hour.

3. Complete column D in a similar fashion to column B. In this case, the previous hour's customer count should be subtracted from the current hour's customer count to determine the customers per hour.

4. Divide column B by column D to determine column E, "Average Check."

5. Add the hourly sales in column B to determine the total daily sales. Add the hourly customer counts in column D to determine the total daily customers. Divide the total of column B by the total of column D to determine the total of column E, the daily average check.

6. Calculate the number of man-hours scheduled per hour from the staffing schedule, and enter it in column F. (A completed staffing schedule,

figure 17B, is included.) Count in increments of one-quarter hour the number of work hours being used in each operating hour. A person scheduled to work 8:30 to 1:00 works one-half hour in the 8:00 to 9:00 hour and one hour in each additional hour.

7. Calculate the customers served per man-hour by dividing the entries in column C by the entries in column F.
8. Calculate the sales per man-hour by dividing the entries in column B by the entries in column F.
9. Add column F to determine the total daily man-hours. Divide this total into the total of column C and into the total of column B to determine the daily customers per man-hour and the daily sales per man-hour, respectively.

The same form, Cash Register Sales Analysis, should be used to complete the weekly composite. The hourly sales (column B) should be added for each day, each hour.

An hourly entry should be made on the composite in column B, "Hourly Sales." The same should be done for column D, "Hourly Customer Count," and column F, "Man-hours." The composite should now be completed as each daily form was, following the instructions in numbers 4, 5, 7, and 8.

Columns B, D, E, G, and H should then be reviewed. Particular attention should be given to the hours of operation in which the hourly figures are lower than the hourly averages at the bottom of columns E, G, and H. These figures may be an indication of opportunities to increase the participation and/or the average check through strategic marketing or promotional activities. Now, notes should be made of the activities to be pursued. This step is now complete.

Figure 17A.
Cash Register Sales Analysis

Operation Name Medical Center Cafeteria   Date 2/21/82

Time	A Hourly Sales Reading	B Hourly Sales	C Customer Count	D Hourly Customer Count	E Average Check	F Man-Hours	G Customers Served per Man-Hour	H Sales per Man-Hour
a.m.								
6:00	0	0	0	0	0	0	0	0
7:00	34.41	34.41	111	111	.31	4.75	23.4	7.25
8:00	59.49	25.08	187	76	.33	5.0	15.2	5.01
9:00	109.32	49.83	367	180	.28	5.5	32.7	9.06
10:00	220.92	111.60	646	279	.40	7.0	39.8	15.94
11:00	334.65	113.73	869	223	.51	7.75	28.7	14.68
p.m.								
12:00	744.78	410.13	1310	441	.93	11.0	40.1	37.28
1:00	1317.45	572.67	1877	567	1.01	11.0	51.5	52.06
2:00	1551.53	234.08	2156	279	.84	10.75	25.9	21.77
3:00	1566.02	14.49	2201	45	.32	8.25	5.5	1.76
4:00	1589.58	23.56	2277	76	.31	7.0	10.8	3.37
5:00	1608.48	18.90	2319	42	.45	7.0	6.0	2.70
6:00	1910.39	301.91	2631	312	.97	5.5	56.7	54.89
7:00	2087.36	176.97	2816	185	.96	4.75	38.9	37.25
8:00	Closed	—	—	—	—	1.0	—	—
9:00	Closed	—	—	—	—	1.0	—	—
10:00	2097.58	10.22	2836	20	.51	2.0	10.0	5.11
11:00	2115.04	17.46	2870	34	.51	2.0	17.0	8.73
a.m.								
12:00	2152.44	37.40	2919	49	.76	2.0	24.5	18.70
1:00	2177.09	24.65	2957	38	.65	2.0	19.0	12.32
2:00	2195.99	18.90	2986	29	.65	2.0	14.5	9.45
3:00	2212.52	16.53	3017	31	.53	2.0	15.5	8.27
4:00	2221.12	8.90	3045	28	.31	1.5	18.6	5.73
5:00	2224.43	3.31	3060	15	.22	1.0	15.0	3.31
6:00	Closed	—	—	—	—	1.25	—	—
Total		2224.43	xxxx	3060	.727	113.0	27.1	19.69
		B		D	E	F	G	H

Figure 17B.
Sample Staffing Schedule

Work Area ___Cafeteria___

Name	Position	Monday	Tuesday	Wednesday	Thursday	Friday	Saturday	Sunday	Hrs
	Supervisor	9-5:30	9-5:30	9-5:30	9-5:30	Off	Off	9-5:30	40.0
	Supervisor	Off	8:30-5	8:30-5	8:30-5	8:30-5	8:30-5	Off	40.0
	Hot line	10:30-7	10:30-7	10:30-7	10:30-7	10:30-7	Off	Off	40.0
	Hot line	10:30-7	10:30-7	10:30-7	10:30-7	10:30-7	10:30-7	Off	40.0
	Hot line	Off	12:00-7	Off	Off	12:00-7	Off	10:30-7	29.0
	Deli	6-2:30	6-2:30	6-2:30	6-2:30	Off	Off	6-2:30	40.0
	Deli	3-7:00	Off	3-7:00	3-7:00	6-2:30	10:30-7	10:30-7	36.0
	Salad bar	6-2:30	Off	Off	6-2:30	5:15-1:45	5:15-1:45	5:15-1:45	40.0
	Salad bar	Off	6-2:30	10:30-7	10:30-7	6-2:30	10:30-7	Off	40.0
	Desserts	10:30-7	6-2:30	6-2:30	6-2:30	Off	Off	10:30-7	40.0
	Desserts	6-2:30	Off	6-2:30	Off	6-2:30	6-2:30	Off	32.0
	Grill	5:15-1:45	5:15-1:45	5:15-1:45	5:15-1:45	Off	Off	5:15-1:45	40.0
	Cashier	Off	10:15-6:45	10:15-6:45	10:15-6:45	10:15-6:45	10:15-6:45	Off	40.0
	Cashier	6:15-2:45	6:15-2:45	6:15-2:45	6:15-2:45	Off	Off	6:15-2:45	40.0
	Cashier	10:15-6:45	10:30-7	Off	Off	6:15-2:45	6:15-2:45	10:15-6:45	40.0
	Midnight leader	7-3:30	7-3:30	7-3:30	7-3:30			7-3:30	
	Midnight cashier	Off	9-5:30	9-5:30	9-5:30	7-3:30	7-3:30	Off	40.0
	Midnight deli	9-5:30	9-5:30	Off	Off	9-5:30	9-5:30	9-5:30	40.0

CHAPTER 18
FOOD COST ANALYSIS

In this section of the audit, the food service administrator will review current food costing practices and portioning procedures, and will make some tentative decisions on whether food cost objectives are being met at current pricing levels. Many operations have much of this information in a cafeteria operations manual. The purposes of this section are as follows:

- To determine the current actual food cost for each item
- To establish the amount of money that the sale of an individual item will generate to pay for fixed costs
- To verify the accuracy of planned costs by comparing them with actual costs
- To reevaluate items that need to be reviewed because they do not meet cost objectives

For the purposes of this study, food cost is defined as the cost of all food items needed to make a product saleable to the customer. These food items include the basic recipe ingredients, condiments, sauces, garnishes, and extras that might enhance sales activity. The following are examples of total food costs:

Cheeseburger

3-oz hamburger	$.33
Hamburger roll	.03
½-oz slice of cheese	.05
1 ketchup (unit portion)	.02
2 pickle slices	.01
Total food cost	$.44

Small tossed salad

3-oz basic salad mix	$.05
2 slices cucumber	.02
1 cherry tomato	.03
Red onion garnish	.01
1-oz salad dressing	.05
Total food cost	$.16

Quiche (Makes 96 portions)

Cream cheese	$7.28
Half & half cream	1.00
Fresh eggs	3.08
Salt	.05
Pepper	.05

Dry mustard	.05
Swiss cheese	7.48
Pie shells	3.00
Total recipe cost	$21.99
Food cost per portion	$ .23

In determining food cost, it is important to know the total cost. In the case of the salad, the dressing costs as much as the basic mix. When the food service administrator makes sound pricing decisions based on accurate food costs, the chance for success is excellent. Such decisions are fair to customers and to the food service administrator as well.

Items currently on the menu should be listed on the Food Cost Analysis sheet (figure 18A). It will be easier if this is done by category—beverage, sandwich, dessert, entree, salad, and so forth, than if it is done randomly. Column 2 is completed by using current menu item portions.

Total food cost should be entered in column 3, and current selling prices in column 4.

Column 5 shows the percentage of the total selling price that is food cost. Column 5 is obtained by dividing column 3 by column 4.

Column 6 is the amount of money that each item in column 1 contributes to operating overhead (fixed costs plus variable nonfood costs). Column 6 is obtained by subtracting column 3 from column 4.

When the first six columns are complete, this portion of the audit is done. Column 7 should be completed for those items that do not meet guidelines and that may require change during action planning. Items with the following characteristics may be considered for change:

- Portion control is not consistent with policy
- Food cost exceeds overall objective
- High price is causing poor sales (Is the high price appropriate?)
- Contribution to overhead is less than 5 cents

Figure 18A.
Food Cost Analysis

				DATE	2/1/82	
1	**2**	**3**	**4**	**5**	**6**	**7**
Item	Portion	Food Cost, $	Sell Price, $	Food Cost, %	Contribution	Change
Soup, large	10 oz	.22	.50	44.0	.280	
Soup, small	5 oz	.11	.30	36.0	.190	
Chowder, large	10 oz	.33	.80	41.3	.470	
Chowder, small	5 oz	.165	.45	36.7	.285	
Hamburger	3 oz	.390	.70	55.8	.310	
Cheeseburger	3 oz + 1 oz	.440	.80	55	.360	
Clamburger	2½ oz	.270	.70	38.6	.430	
Hot dog	10/1	.18	.45	40.0	.270	
Tuna salad sandwich	#16 scoop	.38	.75	50.7	.370	
Egg salad sandwich	#16 scoop	.22	.50	44.0	.280	
Ham sandwich	2 oz	.39	.80	48.8	.410	
Ham & cheese sandwich	2 oz + ½	.44	.90	48.9	.460	
Milk, whole	9 oz	.118	.25	47.2	.132	
Milk, skim	9 oz	.109	.25	43.6	.141	
Milk, chocolate	9 oz	.112	.25	44.8	.138	
Soda, small	9 oz	.040	.25	16.0	.210	
Soda, medium	12 oz	.053	.30	17.7	.247	
Soda, large	16 oz	.071	.35	20.3	.279	
Coffee, small	6 oz	.061	.15	40.7	.089	
Coffee, large	10 oz	.110	.25	44.0	.140	
Fresh fruit	1 piece	.140	.30	46.7	.160	
Pastry	2 oz	.152	.25	60.8	.098	
Potato chips	1 oz	.075	.15	50.0	.075	
Yogurt	8 oz	.260	.40	65.0	.140	

CHAPTER 19
PRODUCT MOVEMENT STUDY

This study deals with how products are selling in relation to total sales and to each other. At its completion, food service administrators will have a good understanding of what their customers want and are willing to pay for. Often, a food service administrator will be able to delete some items from the menu based on information on low-volume sellers identified here. The following are goals for this study:

- Annual unit sales for each menu item
- Annual dollar sales for each menu item
- Percentage of total sales for each item
- Determination of actual food cost objective established by product sales mix
- A best-seller list (the top 20)

The first step in this study is to develop a data base from current sales. There are two ways to do this.

1. A data-capturing cash register that breaks down sales by menu items can save a great deal of time. The data-capturing cash register can be programmed to provide a complete weekly sales analysis, including the number sold of each item and the total dollar revenue of each item. For example, in figure 19A, 1,418 coffees were sold, and the total revenue for coffee was $354.50. Unit sales should be recorded for each item for a one-week to two-week period.

2. Food service administrators who do not have a data-capturing register should proceed in the following manner: Data should be initially recorded on the Menu Item Sales Tally, figure 19B, not the Product Movement Study, figure 19C. All menu items should be entered in column 1, in the same order used for the Food Cost Analysis, figure 18A. Either paid or volunteer help may be needed for the next step of entering the number of items sold on the tally sheet. For each transaction during the study period, each individual item purchased should be recorded. This should be done for at least two days, with seven to 10 days preferred if volunteer help is available. If only two days are used, preference should be given to weekdays. For example, for a purchase that included a hamburger, french fries, a small milk and an apple, a check mark needs to be made next to each of these items on the tally sheet. At the end of the study period, a total unit sales for each item should be tabulated. The difficult part is now over.

On the Product Movement Study (figure 19C), the menu items in column 1 should be entered in the same order as on the Food Cost Analysis, figure 18A.

The food cost percentage from column 5 of the Food Cost Analysis should be entered in column 8 of the Product Movement Study (figure 19C). From column 4 of the Food Cost Analysis, the price of each item should be entered in column 2 of the Product Movement Study.

From the tally sheets (figure 19B), the total number of each item sold over the period of time in the study should be entered in column 3 of the Product Movement Study.

The total number of study days should be entered at the top of figure 19C, and this number should be divided into the total number of operating days, as in the top right corner of the completed Product Movement Study. The result of this division is the factor for all of column 6. The rest of the work is arithmetic, as in figure 19C.

1. Column 4 = column 2 x column 3
2. Column 5 = individual items in column 4 ÷ total of column 4
3. Column 7 = column 4 x column 6
4. Column 9 = column 7 x column 8
5. Total columns 7 and 9

The column 9 total divided by the column 7 total equals a weighted annualized food cost for the operation, the percentage that food cost is of the total dollar sales.

The weighted annualized food cost percentage, 43.5% in figure 19C, is the figure that should be used in calculating overall pricing structures and the break-even point. This is also the figure that should be expected in weekly or monthly sales reports. Any deviation should be reviewed carefully, as this indicates that the cafeteria is not attaining its financial targets.

Figure 19A.
Sales, by Product, Dollars, and Units

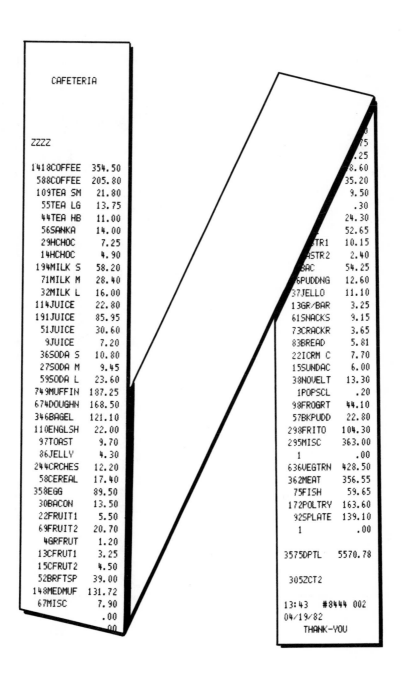

```
        CAFETERIA


ZZZZ

1418COFFEE  354.50
 588COFFEE  205.80
 109TEA SM   21.80
  55TEA LG   13.75
  44TEA HB   11.00
  56SANKA    14.00
  29HCHOC     7.25
  14HCHOC     4.90
 194MILK S   58.20
  71MILK M   28.40
  32MILK L   16.00
 114JUICE    22.80
 191JUICE    85.95
  51JUICE    30.60
   9JUICE     7.20
  36SODA S   10.80
  27SODA M    9.45
  59SODA L   23.60
 749MUFFIN  187.25
 674DOUGHN  168.50
 346BAGEL   121.10
 110ENGLSH   22.00
  97TOAST     9.70
  86JELLY     4.30
 244CRCHES   12.20
  58CEREAL   17.40
 358EGG      89.50
  30BACON    13.50
  22FRUIT1    5.50
  69FRUIT2   20.70
   4GRFRUT    1.20
  13CFRUT1    3.25
  15CFRUT2    4.50
  52BRFTSP   39.00
 148MEDMUF  131.72
  67MISC      7.90
              .00
              .00
```

```
                    0
                   75
                  .25
                 8.60
                35.20
                 9.50
                  .30
                24.30
                52.65
      STR1      10.15
      ASTR2      2.40
      BAC       54.25
     6PUDDNG    12.60
    37JELLO     11.10
    13GR/BAR     3.25
    61SNACKS     9.15
    73CRACKR     3.65
    83BREAD      5.81
    22ICRM C     7.70
    15SUNDAC     6.00
    38NOVELT    13.30
     1POPSCL      .20
    98FROGRT    44.10
    57BKPUDD    22.80
   298FRITO    104.30
   295MISC     363.00
     1            .00
   636VEGTRN    428.50
   362MEAT      356.55
    75FISH       59.65
   172POLTRY    163.60
    32SPLATE    139.10
     1            .00


  3575DPTL     5570.78


   305ZCT2


  13:43   #8444 002
  04/19/82
      THANK-YOU
```

Figure 19B.
Menu Item Sales Tally

	Number of study days _____ 2 _____			

1 Menu item	Day 1	Day 2	Total
Soup, large	LH1 LH1 LH1 ///	LH1 LH1 LH1	33
Soup, small	LH1 LH1 LH1 LH1 LH1 ///	LH1 LH1 LH1 LH1 ///	51
Chowder, large	LH1 LH1 LH1 LH1 LH1 LH1 LH1 /	LH1 LH1 ///	49
Chowder, small	LH1 LH1 LH1 LH1 LH1 LH1	LH1 LH1 LH1 LH1 LH1 /	56
Hamburger	LH1 LH1 LH1 LH1 LH1 LH1 LH1 LH1 LH1 LH1 ///	LH1 LH1 LH1 LH1 LH1 LH1 LH1 LH1 LH1 LH1 LH1 //	110
Cheeseburger	LH1 LH1 LH1 LH1 LH1 LH1 LH1 LH1 LH1 LH1 ////	LH1 LH1 LH1 LH1 LH1 LH1 LH1 LH1 //	96

Figure 19C.
Product Movement Study

Number of Study Days ___2___

Column 6 is determined by dividing your total number of operating days by the number of days in your study.
Ex: 365 operating days ÷ 7 days in study = 52)

1	2	3	4	5	6	7	8	9
Menu Item	Price	# Sold	$ Volume	% of Sales	Factor	Annual $ Volume	Food Cost, %	Annual Food Cost, $
Soup, large	.50	33	16.50	1.2 %	182.5	3011.25	44 %	1324.95
Soup, small	.30	51	15.30	1.2 %	182.5	2792.25	36.7 %	1024.76
Chowder, large	.80	49	39.20	2.9%	182.5	7154.00	41.3%	2954.60
Chowder, small	.45	56	25.20	1.9 %	182.5	4599.00	36.7%	1687.33
Hamburger	.70	110	77.00	5.7%	182.5	14052.50	55.8%	7841.30
Cheeseburger	.80	96	76.80	5.7%	182.5	14016.00	55 %	7708.80
Clamburger	.70	84	58.80	4.3%	182.5	10731.00	38.6%	4142.17
Hot dog	.45	123	55.35	4.1%	182.5	10101.38	40%	4040.55
Tuna salad	.75	130	97.50	7.2%	182.5	17793.75	50.7%	9021.43
Egg salad	.50	124	62.00	4.6%	182.5	11315.00	44.0%	4978.60
Ham sandwich	.80	36	28.80	2.1%	182.5	5256.00	48.8%	2564.93
Ham + cheese sandwich	.90	44	39.60	2.9%	182.5	7227.00	48.9%	3534.00
Milk, whole	.25	402	100.50	7.4%	182.5	18341.35	47.2%	8657.07
Milk, skim	.25	393	98.25	7.2%	182.5	17930.62	43.6%	8689.75
Milk, chocolate	.25	47	11.75	.9%	182.5	2144.38	44.8%	960.68
Soda, small	.25	428	107.00	7.9%	182.5	19527.50	16.0%	3124.40
Soda, medium	.30	301	90.30	6.7%	182.5	16479.75	17.7%	2916.91
Soda, large	.35	122	42.70	3.2%	182.5	7792.75	20.3%	1581.93
Coffee, small	.15	72	10.80	.8%	182.5	1971.00	40.7%	802.20
Coffee, large	.25	165	41.25	3.1%	182.5	7528.13	44.0%	3312.38
Fresh fruit	.30	283	84.90	6.3%	182.5	15494.25	46.7%	7235.82
Pastry	.25	341	85.25	6.3%	182.5	15558.13	60.8%	9459.34
Potato chips	.15	145	21.75	1.6%	182.5	3969.38	50%	1984.69
Yogurt	.40	197	78.80	5.8%	182.5	14381.00	65%	9347.65
			$1,365.30			249,167.27	43.5%	108,896.24

CHAPTER 20
TRANSACTION ANALYSIS

The purpose of the transaction analysis is to clarify the market segmentation study further and to offer new information, both qualitative and quantitative, with regard to specific markets. Once it is complete, food service administrators will be able to determine more specifically the customers now being served and what they are buying, so that similar customers not currently being served can be attracted. In addition, a customer profile can be established by market segment, including typical items purchased and average check.

Transaction analysis is another simple but time-consuming process. As with the product movement study, food service administrators may wish to hire someone to tally this analysis for them, as it should be done for two to three complete days to give proper perspective.

At the top of the Transaction Analysis form, figure 20A, there is a space to indicate time or meal. It is important to isolate studies by meal period and to indicate these meal periods here. Usual combinations are breakfast, lunch, snack, and dinner. Others might include coffee break and midnight supper if the cafeteria has a large volume. Once again, this study must be tailored to the cafeteria operation.

The next section is segment code. The same market segments should be used as were used to identify customers in the survey discussed in chapter 17.

Each market segment should be assigned a letter code. This code will facilitate the tabulation process.

An important decision for the tabulation process is the study interval, which determines which customers' checks will be surveyed. The simple solution is to study all checks, but this could be very tedious for the tabulator. Most persons choose to study every other, or every third, customer. Some go as high as every fourth or every fifth. The number of people served should determine the number studied. Whatever study interval is selected should be used throughout the study. This will eliminate personal selection of customers by the tabulator and will thus maintain accuracy if every customer is not surveyed.

The tabulator should be placed in such a way that he or she has a firm writing surface and can see the customer's tray and the cash register.

For each customer checked, the tabulator needs to enter the correct segment code for the customer, check the "Items Purchased" boxes that apply and enter the total dollar value of the transaction at the bottom of the form. Some of the categories under "Items Purchased" may need to be altered for a specific cafeteria. The *type* of item purchased should be checked, not what was actually purchased. The transaction total should be in dollars and cents.

The tabulator should continue this process until the end of that meal period. At the beginning of a new period, a new transaction analysis sheet and a new study should be begun.

At the end of the day, the transaction tally should be completed for each sheet in the following way:

- *Segment total.* The total number of customers on that sheet from each market segment should be entered here.
- *Average check.* All of the checks for a given segment should be totaled and divided by the total number for that segment.
- *Percentage buying.* The total number of each type of item purchased for each segment should be completed and divided by the total number in that segment. This percentage will represent the number of times an item will be purchased out of 100 purchases by a given segment.

Once all of the individual sheets have been completed for the duration of the study, they should be separated by meal period. The following steps should be taken:

1. The average "average check" should be computed for each segment by totaling all average checks for a segment and dividing by the total number of average checks for that segment.

2. For each segment, the items under "Percentage buying" should be put in order from highest to lowest percentage. The average percentage for each item in each segment during a meal period should be used. For example, in figure 20A, for segment B-Administration, the order would be BEV 100%; SAL 66.7%; ENT 66.3%; SAND, DESS, FRUIT 33.3% each.

3. Finally, a customer buying profile should be completed for each segment by meal period. There is no set format for this. One way that works well is the following:

CUSTOMER PROFILE FOR NURSES

	Breakfast	Lunch	Dinner	Snack
Average Check	$.35	$.85	$1.10	$.35
ITEMS PUR-CHASED	Beverage 80% Snack 65% Entree 15%	Beverage 75% Sandwich 40% Entree 30% Salad 30% Soup 20% Snack 15% Dessert 10%	Beverage 80% Entree 55% Salad 30% Sandwich 15% Dessert 10%	Beverage 90% Snack 65% Dessert 15%

Food service administrators can refer to these profiles when they begin to focus on increasing business during a particular part of the day. They will then be able to direct their marketing programs at the specific markets they want to attract with items those markets are known to purchase.

Figure 20A.
Transaction Analysis

Date 2/15/82

Time or Meal _Lunch_

Segment Code:

A — Nursing
B — Administration
C — Physicians
D — Service Employees
E —
F —
G —
H —

Study Interval — 1 2 ③ 4 5

Transaction Tabulation

Customer No.	1	2	3	4	5	6	7	8	9	10	11	12	13	14	15	16	17	18	19	20	21	22	23	24	25
Code	A	A	A	D	D	A	A	B	D	C	A	D	D	A	B	A	A	C	A	C	B	D	A	D
Items Purchased																									
Snack	X																X								
Beverage	X	X	X	X	X	X	X	X	X	X	X	X	X	X	X	X	X		X	X	X	X	X	X	X
Entree								X		X											X	X		X	
Sandwich	X	X	X			X	X		X		X		X		X		X		X	X			X		X
Salad						X	X	X						X	X		X	X			X				
Soup			X	X												X			X						
Dessert		X			X				X	X	X			X					X	X	X				
Other: Fruit														X								X			
Check Total	1.05	1.37	1.26	.69	58	1.26	1.35	1.65	1.58	1.43	1.68	.65	1.10	1.35	1.80	.53	1.48	1.10	1.25	2.00	2.25	1.45	1.00	1.50	.95

Transaction Tally, % Buying

Segment	Total	Avg. Check	Snack	Bev	Ent	Sand	Sal	Soup	Dess	Fruit
A	12	1.328	16.7	91.7	8.4	66.7	33.4	25.	25.	8.4
B	3	1.634	—	100.	66.3	33.3	66.7	—	33.3	33.3
C	3	1.644	—	33.3	66.3	33.3	33.4	—	100.	—
D	7	.936	—	100.	—	57.2	14.3	33.4	66.7	—
E										
F										
G										
H										

CHAPTER 21
COMPETITION EVALUATION
AND PRICING ANALYSIS

Many of the changes and innovations in the food service industry today are simply modifications of another restaurant's success or elimination of their failures. This applies to hospital food service cafeterias as well. The food service administrator can learn from the competition, be it a local variety store, a chain fast-food restaurant, or diner, or whatever.

This learning process will test observation skills and actually can be fun if done in the right frame of mind. Food service administrators should consider themselves students, not spies.

Competitors' operations to be surveyed should be selected from two sources:
- Those mentioned in the survey
- Those known to be frequented by customers

A list of all competitors should be made and then cut to a maximum of six to eight. Cutting this list should be done by consideration of proximity to the hospital and/or the number of the hospital cafeteria's customers who visit the competition. The surveys done in chapter 16 should be checked to learn where hospital cafeteria customers are going. If there aren't more than two or three competitors, the surveyer should not create them. When the competitor's operation is visited, a survey sheet should be taken along so that nothing is missed. The surveyer should visit that operation when hospital cafeteria customers would. The surveyer should try to be quick and efficient and at the same time to complete the Competition Evaluation and Pricing Analysis, figure 21A.

In the menu items section (column 1) the 10 best-sellers should be determined, if possible. The competition has low-volume items too, and there is no sense spending time on these. Portion size is very important. If they are offering *and* selling larger beverages than the hospital cafeteria is, then it probably could do the same. If they sell a smaller portion of french fries than the hospital cafeteria does but at the same price, then the hospital cafeteria may want to reduce its portion.

When columns 1 through 3 are completed, the entire operation should be examined. Strengths and weaknesses should be reviewed objectively. It is important to remember that the competitor's strength may be a weakness of the hospital cafeteria.

Items to think about as strengths include the following:
- Value pricing—lower cost per ounce on larger items

- Combination pricing—combination costs less than sum of individual items
- Pleasing decor
- Pleasant attitude of employees
- Accessibility of napkins, silverware, and so forth
- Speed through line
- Availability of seats
- Type of service—server, cafeteria, fast-food

Items to think about as weaknesses include these:

- Poor sanitation
- Long lines
- Low quality of food

When columns 1 through 5 are completed, things that should be done as a result of the competition evaluation should be listed in column 6. As many items as come to mind should be listed; the list can be cut later. The next time a change is needed or desired in the cafeteria, this list should be consulted. It is a list of proven winners.

Figure 21A.
Competition Evaluation and Pricing Analysis

Your Operation ___Medical Center Cafeteria___ Date __2/12/82__

| 1 | 2 | 3 | 4 | 5 | 6 |

Competitor: ___Joe's Deli___ Date Visited __2/12/82__

Menu Item	Sell Price	Portion	Strengths	Weaknesses	Opportunities
Hot corned beef	1.75	3 oz	Free pickles on tables	Long lines	Bigger sandwiches for more contribution
Hot roast beef	1.75	3 oz		No tables to sit at	
Pastrami	1.75	3 oz	Fast service		
Joe burger	1.50	2 2-oz on subroll	Sandwiches are bigger than ours		Market our less expensive coffee
Potato salad	.20	2 oz			
Cole slaw	.20	2 oz			
Fruit plate	1.65	6 oz			
Cold beef plate	1.95	3-oz beef 2-oz pot sal.			
Soda	.40	12 oz			
Coffee	.35	8 oz			

Competitor: ___McDougals___ Date Visited __2/11/82__

Menu Item	Sell Price	Portion	Strengths	Weaknesses	Opportunities
Bigger burger	1.45	2 1½-oz loaded	Burger fast-food operation	Limited menu	Review soda pricing
¼-Pounder	1.25	4 oz			
Hamburger	.45	1.5 oz			Possibly reduced size of our burger
Cheeseburger	.55	1.5 oz			
Large french fries	.60	3 oz			
Small french fries	.45	1.8 oz			
Fish sandwich	.75	2½ oz			
Apple pie	.40	2 oz			
Cherry pie	.40	2 oz			
Soda, small	.40	12 oz			
Soda, medium	.50	16 oz			
Soda, large	.60	20 oz			
Coffee	.40	8 oz			

CHAPTER 22
BREAK-EVEN ANALYSIS

Break-even analysis is an accounting process widely used in business to determine at what level of sales an operation will pay for all of its costs—fixed, variable, and semivariable.

Because this figure is determined by using actual expenses from a given business, it is generally accepted as a meaningful decision-making tool. Once established, it gives the food service administrator a guidepost to evaluate the effectiveness of putting plans into action.

Knowledge of break-even is helpful in these areas:

- If a hospital cafeteria is losing money or is subsidized, once break-even is determined, the food service administrator can understand and act on narrowing the gap between break-even and current sales.
- Sales goals can be set based on the amount of profit required over break-even. In subsidy situations, sales goals can be set at the allowable subsidy level.
- Where performance is not running true to budget projections, a review of the break-even analysis can usually pinpoint the area of difficulty for further study.

To begin the break-even analysis, the following definitions are essential:

- *Fixed costs* (FC) are those costs that do not change in direct proportion to sales increases. Examples of fixed costs are costs for rent, utilities, equipment, and janitorial expense. Fixed costs are generally expressed in actual dollars expended or budgeted.
- *Semivariable costs* (SVC) are costs that change at certain levels of sales. The most typical semivariable cost is labor. For example, it may require four persons to operate a basic cafeteria unit that does $100,000 in sales. It may then take one additional person to accomplish each $50,000 in additional sales. In calculating break-even, semivariable costs are treated as fixed costs. Should the semivariable costs change after the break-even is established, it is necessary to recalculate the break-even. Semivariable costs are generally expressed in dollars.
- *Variable costs* (VC) are those costs that change in direct proportion to sales increases or decreases. Examples of variable costs are costs for food, paper, and soap or chemicals. When calculating break-even, variable costs are calculated as a percentage of sales.

The formula for determining the break-even point is:

FC + SVC + VC% = break-even

There is no provision made for profit in the break-even formula. Only costs are utilized in determining break-even. In chapter 11, for example, figure 11A, Cafeteria Operating Statement, January 1980, lists the following costs:

Fixed costs:	
Housekeeping	$400
Utilities	148
Total fixed costs	$548
Semivariable costs:	
Labor	$21,762
Total semivariable costs	$21,762
Variable costs:	
Food cost	$26,668
Paper cost	2,487
Soap or chemicals	112
Miscellaneous	239
Total variable costs	$29,506

With sales of $52,337, variable costs are 56.4% of sales.

Putting these figures into the break-even formula:

1. FC + SVC + VC% = 100% break-even
2. 548 + 21,762 + 56.4% = 100% break-even
3. 548 + 21,762 = 100% - 56.4%
4. 22,310 = 43.6% break-even
5. 22,310 ÷ 43.6% = break-even
6. $51,170 = break-even

In other words, $51,170 will pay all operating costs but will result in no profit or loss.

Figure 22A, Break-even Calculation, provides the steps necessary for determining break-even. Food service administrators should work through this calculation twice, the first time using annual *budget* figures and the second time *actual cost* figures.

For the second calculation, the current actual variable cost percentage of sales should be used, as well as actual fixed cost and semivariable cost figures. In the middle of an accounting year, the break-even year to date should be calculated. Then, a full-year projection based on the year to date must be made.

When the two calculations have been completed, actual and budget break-even figures should be compared. If there is a substantial difference between budget break-even and actual break-even figures, the following items should be examined:

- Pricing: Is it current and correct?
- Waste: Is it more than planned?
- Rip-off: Can it be controlled?
- Cafeteria employee meals: Are they according to policy?
- Pricing formulas: Can these goals be achieved?   Any of these areas that are problems should be included in the food service administrator's action plan.

Figure 22A.
Break-Even Calculation

To calculate break-even, determine:
- Annual sales
- Variable costs
- Fixed costs
- Semivariable costs

Use *annual budget* figures the first time and *actual cost* figures the second time.

Break-Even

Annual sales: $ _____

Variable costs: $ _____

_____

_____

Total variable costs $ _____

Variable costs as a
percentage of sales: _____ %

Semivariable costs: $ _____

_____

_____

Total semivariable costs: $ _____

Fixed costs: _____

_____

Total fixed costs: $ _____

Follow steps 1 through 6 in the break-even formula to determine break-even.

$$FC + SVC + VC\% = BREAK\text{-}EVEN \ (100\%)$$

CHAPTER 23
AUDIT SUMMARY

Each chapter of the audit is designed to cause food service administrators to look in depth at the various operations within their cafeteria operation. As each chapter is completed, areas can probably be recognized that need to be worked on or where opportunities exist for increased sales, lower costs, or improved service. To complete the audit, then, it is important to list these items for which action should be initiated.

For each chapter of the audit, a list should be made of the items requiring action. For example:

Operations checklist:
- Purchase and install new menu boards.
- Begin a "Specials of the Day" program.
- Take soup off the line and make it self-service. Electric soup pots will be needed for this.

Market survey and segmentation study:
- Consider nursing department request for a salad bar. Nursing is a large market, and a salad bar would be a winner.
- Evaluate why only 10% of the office staff is being served at coffee break.
- Check out Joe's Diner to determine why service staff goes there for lunch.

Cash register sales analysis:
- Work on a marketing program to attract more business between 2:00 p.m. and 4:00 p.m.

Food cost analysis:
- Review sandwich bar for price increases. Food cost is over guideline.
- Check portion control on casserole items. Portions are larger than planned.

Product movement study:
- Prepackaged pastry items are slow sellers. They probably can be eliminated from menu.
- Actual annualized food cost is 51%, 3% higher than our goal of 48%. Verify the reason for this.

Transaction analysis:

- The service employees are heavy meat-and-potato eaters at lunch. Possibly a blue plate special similar to Joe's Diner should be offered to attract them to the cafeteria.
- There is an overall low purchase rate of entrees at breakfast. A marketing plan should be considered to increase their sales or eliminate them.

Competition evaluation:

- A three-size cold beverage program similar to McDougal's should be introduced.
- The Friday fish fry at Joe's Diner appeared to be a big seller.

Break-even analysis:

- The hospital cafeteria is operating at an annual sales rate of $2,600 below break-even. With a goal to achieve break-even, a substantial effort must be developed to reduce food costs as a percentage of sales so that break-even can be reduced by $2,600.

Once the list of items requiring action is completed, a priority rank should be put on each item. This will help with accomplishing the action plan. For example, using the sample list, the food cost analysis and the product movement action would also help accomplish the break-even action, so these two might be priority one. Priority two might be the implementation of the salad bar indicated in the market survey and segmentation study. Each item on the list should be costed out. This process will also help in setting priorities.

CHAPTER 24
METHODOLOGIES
FOR INCREASING PROFITABILITY

In this chapter, some ideas will be reviewed for use in action planning. Most of these ideas are general in nature, providing an opportunity for food service administrators to add the specifics to create a customized program. There are many methods in the marketing process, but the five outlined here are the most commonly used:

- Increasing sales—number of customers
- Increasing sales—amount of average check
- Decreasing variable costs
- Decreasing fixed costs
- Increasing prices

It should be noted that increasing prices is the *last* alternative discussed. Generally, increasing prices has the most negative effect on customers, often decreasing customer volume and/or sales dollars. Other than legitimate pass-through cost increases, price increases should be a last resort as a creative method for increasing profit or attaining break-even.

SALES INCREASE WITH ADDITIONAL CUSTOMERS

1. Increasing market penetration is a good prospect here. Knowledge of individual market preferences has been provided from the audit. Potential sales volume in a market can be determined by multiplying the number of potential customers not being served by that market segment's average check. This should be done for each market, and then a campaign should be directed at those markets with the highest sales potential.
2. Increasing sales efforts during slow periods is another approach. Slow periods should be identified and then a specific marketing plan developed for each. For instance:
   a. *Breakfast*. A full "breakfast special"—two eggs, toast, home fries, and jelly could be offered—value priced at 60% of food cost because fixed costs are already paid. Coffee should not be included because most customers will buy this anyway.
   b. *Morning break*. A "coffee and" promotion could be run, promoting coffee sales with a muffin or doughnut by discounting the combined price by 10 to 20%.
   c. *Afternoon break*. Combination pricing with discounts could be promoted, similar to the one during the morning break.

d. *Midnight special.* Food selections that are appropriate to customers' preferences could be promoted, giving the customers the feeling that their needs are being considered. Because midnight employees are generally soup-eaters, a soup special with additional purchase could be offered.

Repeat business can be encouraged through the use of coupons. Three methods work well:

e. Discount off next purchase of similar item.
f. Buy five and sixth is free. (This is really a 20% discount.)
g. Interest during slow periods can be created by offering a coupon for purchasing an item during a slow period with another purchase. For instance, with every purchase of $1.00 or more at lunch, a coupon could be offered for a free small coffee with purchase of breakfast special.

3. Customers can be attracted from your competition by offering them products or promoting services that now are attracting customers to the competition.
4. Markets not being served should be reviewed. For example, construction workers in the hospital during a renovation or building project are an often overlooked market. These customers generally are hearty eaters with high average checks. Proven marketing campaigns for this market are two sandwiches for the price of one and one-half or a soup, sandwich, and beverage combination.

SALES INCREASE THROUGH INCREASED CHECK AVERAGE

1. Combination pricing works by offering the customer a reduced price when purchasing multiple items. Sample ideas are:
   a. Soup, sandwich, beverage
   b. Soup, salad, beverage
   c. Entree, potato, vegetable
   A general rule of thumb to offer is 10 to 15% discounts in this promotion.
2. Bigger is better. A commonly used marketing tool in fast-food operations, the theory is the bigger an item is, the more money will be contributed to fixed cost or profit even though the food cost percentage increases. For instance, soda costs approximately 1 cent per ounce. A 12-oz cup costs 12 cents and sells for 30 cents, contributing 18 cents at 40% food cost. A 20-oz cup costs 20 cents and sells for 45 cents, contributing 25 cents at 44% food cost. This concept works well for most menu items.
3. Add-on purchases are similar to combination pricing in that the customer is encouraged to buy more. This is generally done by suggestion (Would you like french fries with your hamburger?) or by signs advertising an item being promoted for sale.
4. Impulse buying is effected primarily by access to the item. Items that customers might not normally purchase should be promoted by being placed in areas where customers may wait in line, areas that have high visibility, or areas that precede the purchasing area the customer will use. Desserts first is a common promotion here. Another aid to impulse buying is to use eye-appealing garnishes or line displays.

DECREASING VARIABLE COSTS

1. Items with a lower food cost should be added. One particularly appealing technique here is replacing meat entrees with vegetarian entrees. The demand for vegetarian foods is increasing, and they tend to be less expensive.
2. Emphasis on disposables should be reduced by switching to china and glassware. If the dishwashing capabilities are available, soap is cheaper than plastic.
3. Items with a high food cost should be eliminated. Once the food cost guideline has been determined, it should be allowed to work. If an item doesn't move, it should be removed from the menu.
4. Items totaling 5% of the menu could be eliminated. From the product movement study, the 5% of menu that accounts for the least amount of money should be determined. These items should be taken off the menu, and similar items that remain should be promoted.

DECREASING FIXED COSTS

1. Labor staffing should be consistent with the number of customers being served. Labor reductions through the use of 35-hour or 37.5-hour weeks, part-time employees, or revised schedules should be considered.
2. Operating hours could be reduced. A cost/benefit ratio should be established for hours of operation that have minimal sales. This reduction should be explained to your administrator in terms of dollars that can be saved. Alternatives like vending machines or reduced service should also be suggested.

INCREASING PRICES

If all else has failed, another alternative to creating a more positive balance sheet is to raise prices. The following steps should be considered:

1. How much is needed? The amount of money needed to accomplish this goal must be determined first.
2. The food cost analysis should be rechecked. Are there items that should be repriced because of legitimate cost increases? If so, the increases should be planned and a determination made of how much of the dollar requirements outlined in step 1 will be accomplished by these increases.
3. Next, an incremental price study should be done. The effect in dollars of increasing the top 20 items in the product movement study by 5, 10, or 15 cents should be evaluated. Often, the volume of these items at moderate increases will create the necessary sales dollars. They also are high demand items and are less likely to suffer substantial cuts in purchases.
4. Finally, an across-the-board increase should be considered. The overall percentage increase required should be determined and applied to as many items as necessary to accomplish the goal. Often this increase will need to be applied on an average basis, with some items at a higher percentage and some at a lower percentage.

Price increases are not without substantial problems. Some changes in customer behavior that may occur include:

- An increase in brown bagging
- Trading down, that is, buying smaller or less expensive items than before
- A perceived lowering in the quality of the product and a perceived decrease in value

After these techniques have been reviewed, the food service administrator should select the ones that might help accomplish the goals or needs as outlined in the last section of the audit. The probable dollar impact of each should be determined. Next, the probable effect of each on customer service should be determined. Methodologies should be ranked by probable chance for success. The best ones are generally those that offer customers increased value (perceived or actual) and the operation either increased dollars in profit or reduced loss.

The suggested ideas in this chapter are only samples of what can be done using the information from the eight mini-studies. Each food service administrator should discover many more ways of improving cafeteria operations that are specific to his or her own operation.

CHAPTER 25
DEVELOPING AN OPERATING STRATEGY

In chapters 15 through 24, food service administrators had an opportunity to review the operation in their cafeteria, to identify areas that may require change, and to select potential projects that would strengthen their operation. So that planning and implementing these projects can be begun, some guidelines for establishing priorities are needed. These guidelines will be documented in the operating strategy.

The strategy selected will be determined by two factors:
- Financial objectives
- Service objectives

The attainment of these two sets of objectives simultaneously will require careful negotiation and planning. They can be attained, however, in a single well defined plan that is workable and measurable.

Financial objectives should be set first. This is done primarily to set parameters for service objectives. Financial objectives are best done with the help and support of hospital administration. One of the three objectives listed below should be selected:
- The cafeteria should break even on all operating costs
- The cafeteria should make a profit of _____ %
- The cafeteria will be subsidized from hospital revenue at _____ % of operating costs

Once an objective has been selected, service objectives should be considered. Increases in service objectives generally correlate with increases in costs. The ability to meet service objectives will be affected by the financial objectives.

These service objectives should be reviewed:
- Operating hours
- Menu, both type and number of menu items
- Level of service at a given hour
- Staffing requirements
- Pricing
- Portion and portion control
- Customer needs

Each objective should be defined as completely as possible. These objectives are operating goals. They should be identified specifically so that achievement of the goals can be measured.

Examples of service objectives are the following:
1. Food service available 24 hours a day

     a. Cafeteria open 6:00 a.m. to 6:00 p.m., 8:00 p.m. to midnight
     b. Vending available to service remainder of 24-hour schedule
  2. Lunch menu to include
     a. 2 hot entrees
     b. 6 sandwiches
     c. 6 beverages
     d. 3 salads
     e. 5 desserts (including fresh fruit)
  3. Pricing will attain an average of two times food cost

When service goals have been identified, they should be reviewed to determine whether they have any effect on financial goals and whether modifications are required. Any necessary modifications should then be made.

All of the financial and service objectives should be listed and priorities assigned to these items from most important to least important. The order of financial and service objectives is the decision of the food service administrator and should reflect the hospital's operating policies. The summary of these objectives is the operating strategy for the food service administrator.

CHAPTER 26
ACTION PLANNING

Action planning is the process used to combine the audit, methodology, and strategy portions of the guidelines. Very simply, the action plan is a process for ordering the action to be taken to solve problems identified in the audit. The action taken will be consistent with the priorities set in the strategy plan. Many of the actions will come directly from the methodologies list discussed in chapter 24.

The key steps in action planning are to:
1. Identify and define the problem
2. Select appropriate action and determine measures of success if available
3. Identify those persons who are responsible for implementing the action
4. Set a date for completion of the action step
5. Determine who is responsible for follow-up and review

There are two places where problems or opportunities may have surfaced. One is in the audit and the other is in items in the operating strategy that are not being met. Many of the action steps can be found in the sample methodologies in chapter 24 except for very specific customer requests and some results from the competition survey. On the action planning form, the persons listed as responsible are those persons who are directly responsible for implementation. A reasonable date for implementation should be set. A food service administrator is usually the best person for follow-up and review. Samples of Action Planning, figure 26A, follow as an example.

The action plan is the final step in the audit and marketing process.

The success of the hospital food service cafeteria now rests with the food service administrator.

Figure 26A.
Action Planning Form

Date 01/10/82 Problem	Action	Person Responsible	Date for Completion	Follow-up and Review
Medical Center currently operating at 10% subsidy. Strategy plan calls for break-even by 1983.	Implement the following within 30 days. Review at end of 90 days for probability of attaining goal. Change if necessary. To Increase Sales 1. Breakfast special from 8 a.m. to 10 a.m. 2 eggs, toast, home fries – 79¢ Introduce with coupon for 69¢ given with purchase over $1.00 at lunch 11 a.m. to 1 p.m.	Cafeteria Manager	2/10/82	
	2. Begin a Blue Plate special at lunch – Entree, potato, and vegetable for price of entree and vegetable.	Cafeteria Manager	2/10/82	Food Service Director
	To Reduce Variable Cost 1. Change to china dinner plates and dessert plates to replace paper. Purchase glass racks and glasses to replace plastic cups.	Materials Management	2/10/82	4/10/82
	2. Replace one entree at lunch with one vegetarian entree of lower food cost.	Chef	2/10/82	
Nursing personnel surveyed requested a salad bar.	Request in new capital budget $2,500 for salad bar purchase. Justification: at a food cost of 33% of sales, unit will pay for itself in 2.5 months, after which this item will contribute to lower food cost and satisfy needs of priority segment. Salads to be priced at: Small .50 Medium .90 Large 1.50	Cafeteria Manager Materials Management	10/01/82	Food Service Director
Average check at morning break is only 21.3¢, indicating beverage sales only.	Encourage purchase of coffee and doughnuts with combination pricing. Cost of coffee, cream, sugar, and cup is .075 and selling price is .15. Doughnut cost is .15 and selling price is .30. Selling price for coffee and doughnut combined at .40 increases contribution over sale of coffee alone by .10. Coffee alone: .15–.075 = .075. Coffee plus doughnut: .40–.075–.15 = .175.	Morning Shift Leader	3/15/82	Cafeteria Manager
Sandwich area has no portion control procedure.	1. Establish procedure indicating type of bread to be used, portion size by weight or scoop, lettuce, tomato, cheese, and pickle portions.	Food Service Director	3/1/82	
	2. Purchase scoops.	Materials Management	3/1/82	Cafeteria Manager
	3. Train employees.	Food Service Director/ Cafeteria Manager	3/15/82	
Long lines at cashiers' station at 12 noon.	1. Open 3rd register for one hour.			
	2. Request 1 hour of volunteer time from 12 to 1 in exchange for free lunch.	Food Service Director	4/1/82	
	3. Provide training program for volunteers.	Cafeteria Manager	4/15/82	Cafeteria Manager
	4. Communicate to customers the times when lines are shorter – 1 to 1:30 and 11 to 11:30.	Food Service Director/ Public Relations Department	2/1/82	

REFERENCES

1. *Crest* survey. Cincinnati: Procter and Gamble, 1978.
2. Buchanan, Robert D. Pricing menus for profit. *Food Service Marketing*, March 1977.
3. Patterson, Robert T. How prime costing can maximize profits. *Food Service Marketing*, February 1980.
4. Buchanan, Robert D. Pricing menus for profit. *Food Service Marketing*, April 1977.
5. Galya, Gerald J. Time, motion, and staffing in the dietary department. In: *Productivity Improvements in Hospital Dietary Systems.* Center for Hospital Management Engineering. Chicago: American Hospital Association, 1978.
6. Blanken, Howard M. A time-task allocation method for labor control in hospital food service departments. In: *Productivity Improvements in Hospital Dietary Systems.* Center for Hospital Management Engineering. Chicago: American Hospital Association, 1978.
7. Kaud, Faisal A. Implementing the chilled food concept. *Hospitals, J.A.H.A.* 46:97, Aug. 1972.
8. Ball, Edward W., and Durfee, Kent. Hospital airline galley, does fly. In: *Productivity Improvements in Hospital Dietary Systems.* Center for Hospital Management Engineering. Chicago: American Hospital Association, 1978.
9. Crum, Carole. Health care facility merger: an opportunity for productivity improvement and innovation in the dietary department. In: *Productivity Improvements in Hospital Dietary Systems.* Center for Hospital Management Engineering. Chicago: American Hospital Association, 1978.
10. This format is a variation on the Cashier's Report presented in *Determination and Allocation of Food Service Costs*, American Society for Hospital Food Service Administrators of the American Hospital Association. Chicago: AHA, 1975. That report is a good basis from which to design an individualized cash report for a specific hospital cafeteria.
11. A good summary format to use unchanged or as a basis for an individualized summary form is "Public Feeding Weekly Revenue Report and Meal Count Summary" in *Determination and Allocation of Food Service Costs,* American Society for Hospital Food Service Administrators of the American Hospital Association. Chicago: AHA, 1975.
12. Kaud, Faisal A. In: *Preparation of a Hospital Food Service Department Budget.* American Society for Hospital Food Service Administrators of the American Hospital Association. Chicago: AHA, 1978.

13. Sill, Brian T. Restaurant merchandising for the independent operator. *The Cornell Hotel and Restaurant Administration Quarterly.* Ithaca, NY, May 1980.
14. Wenzel, G. L. *How to Build Volume.* Austin, TX: George L. Wenzel, 1954.

BIBLIOGRAPHY

Aldrich, P. J., and Miller, G. A. *Standardizing Recipes for Institutional Use.* Agricultural Experiment Station Circular Bulletin 233. East Lansing: Michigan State University, 1963.

American Society for Hospital Food Service Administrators of the American Hospital Association. *Determination and Allocation of Food Service Costs.* Chicago: AHA, 1975.

———. *Preparation of a Hospital Food Service Department Budget.* Chicago: AHA, 1978.

Blue Goose, Inc. *The Blue Goose Buying Guide for Fresh Fruits and Vegetables.* Fullerton, CA: Blue Goose, Inc., 1961.

Brodner, J., and others. *Profitable Food and Beverage Operation.* 4th ed. New York: Ahrens Publishing Company, Inc., 1962.

Center for Hospital Management Engineering. *Productivity Improvements in Hospital Dietary Systems.* Chicago: American Hospital Association, 1978.

Dukas, P., and Lundberg, D. E. *How to Operate a Restaurant.* New York: Ahrens Publishing Company, Inc., 1962.

Freshwater, John F. A productivity index for cafeteria workers. *The Cornell Hotel and Restaurant Administration Quarterly.* Ithaca, Y, August 1967.

Kaud, F. A. Implementing the chilled food concept. *Hospitals, J.A.H.A.* 46:97, August 1, 1972.

Keiser, J., and Kallio, E. *Controlling and Analyzing Costs in Food Service Operations.* New York: John Wiley & Sons, Inc., 1974.

Keister, D. C. *How to Increase Profits with Portion Control.* Chicago: National Restaurant Association, 1972.

Levie, A. *The Meat Handbook.* Westport, CT: Avi Publishing Company, Inc., 1963.

Levings, P. *Profit from Foodservice: A Q and A Approach.* Boston: Cahners Publishing Company, Inc., 1974.

Levinson, C. *Food and Beverage Operation.* Englewood Cliffs, NJ: Prentice-Hall, Inc., 1976.

National Association of Meat Purveyors. *Meat Buyer's Guide to Portion Control Meat Cuts.* Chicago: NAMP, July 1972.

———. *Meat Buyer's Guide To Standardized Meat Cuts.* Chicago: NAMP, July 1972.

National Live Stock and Meat Board. *Lessons on Meat.* 2nd ed. Chicago: NLSMB, August 1966.

————. *Meat Evaluation Handbook*. Chicago: NLSMB, 1977.

National Turkey Federation. *Turkey Handbook*. Reston, VA: NTF, 1972.

Peddersen, Raymond B. *SPECS: The Comprehensive Food Service Purchasing & Specification Manual*. Boston: Cahners Books International, Inc., 1977.

Sill, B. T. Restaurant merchandising for the independent operator. *The Cornell Hotel and Restaurant Administration Quarterly*. Ithaca, NY, May 1980.

Stokes, Judy Ford. *Cost-Effective Quality Food Service*. Germantown, MD: Aspen Systems Corp., 1979.

Swift and Company. *Cuts of Meat—How You Can Identify Them*. Agricultural Research Bulletin No. 7. Swift Agricultural Research Dept., Chicago.

U.S. Department of Agriculture. *Institutional Meat Purchase Specifications for Fresh Beef*. Washington, DC: USDA, January 1975.

————. *Institutional Meat Purchase Specifications for Cured, Cured and Smoked, and Fully-Cooked Pork Products*. Series 500. Washington, DC: USDA, June 1971.

————. *Institutional Meat Purchase Specifications for Cured, Dried, and Smoked Beef Products*. Series 600. Washington, DC: USDA, January 1970.

————. *Institutional Meat Purchase Specifications, General Requirements*. Washington, DC: USDA, August 1971.

————. *Institutional Meat Purchase Specifications for Fresh Lamb and Mutton*. Washington, DC: USDA, January 1975.

————. *Institutional Meat Purchase Specifications for Fresh Pork*. Washington, DC: USDA, January 1975.

————. *Institutional Meat Purchase Specifications for Fresh Veal and Calf*. Washington, DC: USDA, July 1975.

Wanderstock, J. J., and Wellington, G. H. *Let's Cut Meat*. New York State College of Agriculture, Cornell Extension Bulletin 1053. Reprinted January 1963.

Wenzel, G. L. *How to Build Volume*. Austin, TX: George L. Wenzel, 1954.

West, B. B., and others. *Food Service in Institutions*. 5th ed. New York: John Wiley & Sons, Inc., 1977.

Wilkinson, Jule, ed. *The Anatomy of Food Service Design 2*. Boston: CBI Publishing Company, Inc., 1978.